T0088118

# KOMBUCHA AND KIMCHI

*For Ella and Esther*

© Text Soki Choi, Photos Roland Persson 2018

First English-language edition
English language translation copyright © 2019, 2021 Skyhorse Publishing
Original title *Kimchi och kombucha: Den nya vetenskapen om hur tarmbakterierna stärker din hjärna*
First published by Bonnier Fakta, Stockholm, Sweden
Published in the English language by arrangement with Bonnier Rights, Stockholm, Sweden

All rights reserved. No part of this book may be reproduced in any manner without the express written consent of the publisher, except in the case of brief excerpts in critical reviews or articles. All inquiries should be addressed to Skyhorse Publishing, 307 West 36th Street, 11th Floor, New York, NY 10018.

Skyhorse Publishing books may be purchased in bulk at special discounts for sales promotion, corporate gifts, fund-raising, or educational purposes. Special editions can also be created to specifications. For details, contact the Special Sales Department, Skyhorse Publishing, 307 West 36th Street, 11th Floor, New York, NY 10018 or info@skyhorsepublishing.com.

Skyhorse® and Skyhorse Publishing® are registered trademarks of Skyhorse Publishing, Inc.®, a Delaware corporation.

Visit our website at www.skyhorsepublishing.com.

10 9 8 7 6 5 4 3 2 1

Library of Congress Cataloging-in-Publication Data is available on file.

Photos by Roland Persson
Graphic design and illustrations by Katy Kimbell
Cover design by Laura Klynstra
Cover photo credit: Roland Persson

Hardcover ISBN: 978-1-5107-4898-9
Paperback ISBN: 978-1-5107-5999-2
Ebook ISBN: 978-1-5107-4899-6

Printed in China

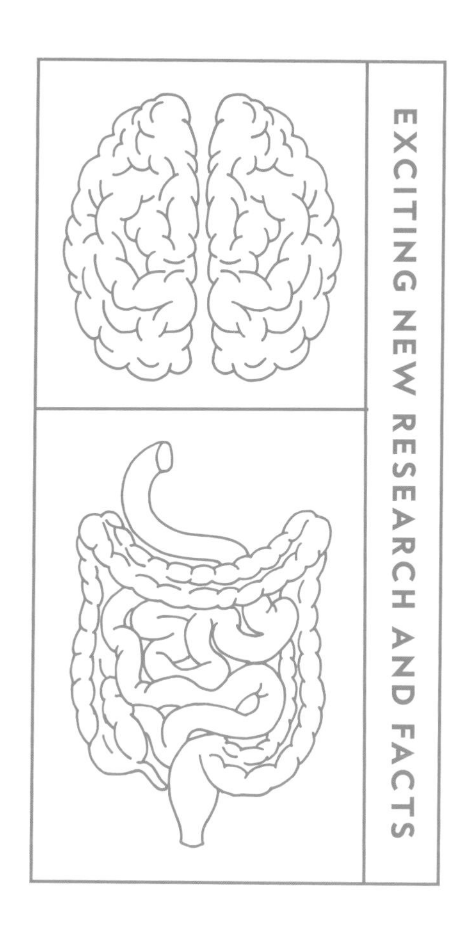


SOKI CHOI

# KOMBUCHA AND KIMCHI

## How Probiotics and Prebiotics Can Improve Brain Function

**Translated by Ellen Hedström**

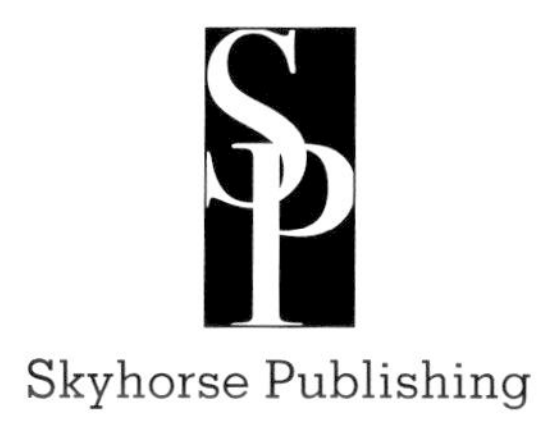

## TABLE OF CONTENTS

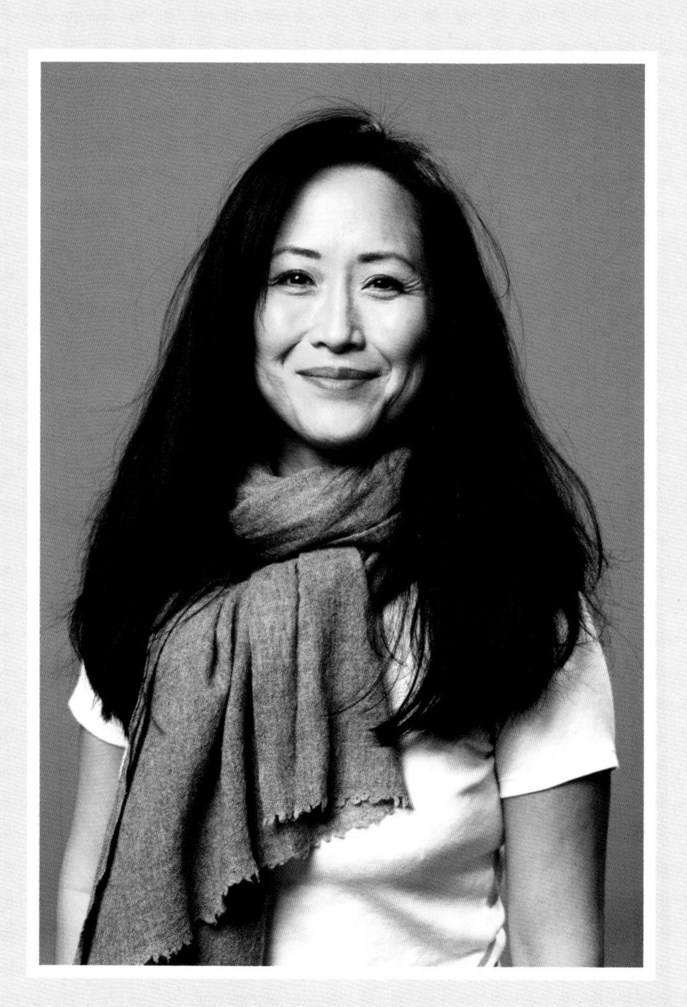

# PROLOGUE

## *The start of a new era*

There is currently a huge buzz around, in many people's opinion, the next big thing in medicine and well-being; the link between gut bacteria and the brain. It seems that gut bacteria don't just play a role in regulating our immune system, but they are also a deciding factor in many issues relating to our mental health. Even if research is still in its infancy, the rapidly expanding output of studies show important links between everything from stress, anxiety, depression, Alzheimer's, Parkinson's, autism, ADHD, and so on, and an imbalance in gut flora.

Not the best news for those who have spent time and energy on self-help books, medicine, psychologists, and other forms of therapy when a simple fecal transplant (a fancy term for stool transfer) would have sufficed.

It seems strange, but also rather amusing, that modern people, who are capable of landing on the moon and splitting the atom, have not researched gut bacteria until now, especially when this busy ecosystem has existed literally right beneath our eyes in our gut—or maybe that's why!

Did you know that there are 39 trillion living microorganisms in your gut? Thirty-nine trillion! I had to double-check the number of zeros: 39,000,000,000,000—that's more than the number of stars in our galaxy. Imagine a huge, sprawling kingdom populated by bacterial strains and other exotic inhabitants such as archaea, protozoa, fungi, and viruses. Together they create a fascinating ecosystem where they play, get along, and sometimes bicker in our furry intestines. I don't exactly envy the existence of the bacteria farther down in the splashy intestinal tubes; it's dark, damp, sour, short-lived, and brutal. So it's no surprise that for a long time our unicellular inhabitants were considered unimportant with only the most basic tasks to complete, such as producing sulfuric gases and feces. The discovery of "gut flora" and its importance to our brain has greatly revised our previous understanding of how disease occurs, and this opens up new possibilities for us to influence our mental health.

In order to equip you with this new knowledge about gut flora's effect on your brain, I have pored over more than four hundred scientific articles (even more than what I had studied for my own PhD). Even more articles were published while I wrote this book, which was challenging, but it also showed how fresh, vibrant, and ever-changing this field of research is. Since I'm not a medical doctor and my own research hasn't focused on gut bacteria and the brain (rather complex medical systems), I asked several fact-checkers to quality assure this text to inspire confidence in my readers. As I wrote, more thoughts and questions arose, and some have been formatted into little boxes I've called "Soki Choi reflects," that are scattered throughout the book.

In this book I will reveal how the gut, gut bacteria, and the brain communicate. I'll also present groundbreaking new research on the relationships between gut bacteria and our most common diagnoses relating to mental health and the brain. First and foremost, I will show you the effect that fiber and bacteria can have on the brain and why this might be the case. In addition to general tips I provide on which foods will strengthen your brain, we will also dive into the magical world of kimchi and kombucha. Both kimchi and kombucha are full of healthy fiber and bacteria and consistently top the charts for the world's healthiest foods. Both are also from my second home country, Korea. Did you know that the people who are thought to live the longest reside in South Korea (where locals eat kimchi every day)? Last but not least, I will give you some of my best recipes for kimchi and kombucha—all to kick-start your brain.

Welcome to the amazing world of bacteria; the adventure starts here . . .

CHAPTER 1

# The microbiotic revolution

# *The brilliance of evolution*

Bacteria can be found everywhere. They live in the deepest seas, the hottest springs, the coldest icy landscapes, and even up in the clouds, where they act as seeds to rain and snow. The live in the mouth, nose, belly button, lungs, breast tissue, genitals, semen, saliva, and of course our gut. Bacteria have and will always be part of our evolutionary history. To understand how essential bacteria are for the survival of humankind, we need to remind ourselves of how life began. So let us raise our eyes to the heavens and rewind to the birth of our universe.

## The rise of bacteria

It can be hard to imagine, but 13.7 billion years ago there was nothing; just total silence, emptiness, and stillness. In one ferocious moment—the big bang—all material, energy, space, and time was created from this empty void. From this gigantic primal explosion our new universe sprung to life and expanded at an enormous rate—even faster than the speed of light. Planet Earth may appear large and unique to us humans, but our blue planet is just a tiny speck of dust in an infinite universe.

In relation to the age of the universe, our home planet is very young. Earth was "only" created 4.5 billion years ago, but even this figure is such a huge amount of time to get to grips with. Let us therefore compress the life span of earth into a year. Imagine that it's Monday, January 1. Your home planet—Earth—doesn't yet have a solid surface. By February an atmosphere is created, which cools and solidifies the earth's surface to a hard crust, then the oceans are created. March is when it all happens: the first signs of life appear in the form of single-celled organisms. During April and May the heat becomes unbearable and it rains all the time. In September the earth is struck by an ice age, making the earth cold, and by October it warms up again. During the fall, multicellular organisms such as fungi and jellyfish appear, and by November fish are created. In December the first vertebrates crawl onto land. In the middle of December the most feared animals, the dinosaurs, dominate our world while the first flowers blossom (to my mother's delight). However, the night of December 26, the earth is struck by an asteroid and in one fell swoop, all dinosaurs disappear from our planet. Instead mammals roam around while the earth constantly changes through weather, wind, volcanic eruptions, and earthquakes. Now we are into the last week of the year and things move fast. Mountain ranges such as the Andes, the Alps, and the Himalayas are created (to the great joy of people like me who love skiing and climbing). Midnight is getting closer, and you may be wondering when humans appeared? Less than 30 minutes before the strike of midnight on New Year's Eve, on December 31, man is finally born and can begin his evolutionary journey on earth (a close call!).

The main point in this short evolutionary tale is to show how for the most part of earth's existence, it was inhabited by tiny bacteria, invisible to our eyes. From March to October there were no other forms of life than our friends, the single-celled organisms. All trees, plants, birds, animals, and insects that you see in nature today are all evolutionary newbies; meanwhile, bacteria lay the foundations for you, your friends and family, and all other life-forms. In the words of an American scientist, "animals are our evolutionary icing but bacteria are the cake itself."

## The world's most important marriage

Of all the fantastic things about the unusual history of microbes, there is one unique deciding factor that needs to be mentioned: the unification between archaea and bacteria. This is without a doubt evolution's largest and most unlikely relationship, and I have chosen to call this event the world's most important marriage. But first we need a quick biology lesson.

All living things can be placed into three groups: eukaryotes, archaea, and eubacteria. In biological terms, humans are eukaryotes, a category that also includes all animals, plants, fungi, and even algae. Prior to the existence of eukaryotes, all living things consisted of either eubacteria or archaea. Bacteria are known to most of us, but few have heard of archaea. Originally, researchers thought that archaea were bacteria because they look similar on the outside; however, they are completely different. Archaea, as opposed to bacteria, like the extreme things in life. They hang out in boiling volcanoes, swim around in corrosive acid, press themselves to the bottom of the deepest seas, splash around in super-salty water, or chill out in the coldest ice blocks. Put it simply, they love extreme sports! During the first 2.5 billion years on earth, archaea and bacteria lived side by side, following their own trajectories. Destiny, however, had other ideas. One day, a bacteria—let's call it Bacterium—was so impressed by the extreme sportsman archaea that it escaped and, in some bizarre way, managed to squeeze in and merge with the archaea. It's through this marriage that scientists believe multicellular eukaryotes came to be, the prerequisite for all life on earth. This is the story of the origin of humankind: two huge domains of unicellular lives, bacteria and archaea, that merged to create a third multicellular life, eukaryotes, to which the human race belongs.

With the principle of "strength in numbers," more eukaryotes started to work with each other and some lumped together to gain more genes and build more elaborate organs and systems. The process eventually led to larger and more complex life-forms being created, such as animals and humans. And while the eyes, the liver, and other organs also evolved later on during independent instances, scientists believe that the birth of the eukaryote cell was and is the most unique and important incident of all. In the context of earth's calendar, the biggest marriage in evolutionary history occurred at the end of October.

## A constantly evolving living ecosystem

The microbiota is a living ecosystem that is constantly changing. It can take care of us or poison us, depending on what we feed it. The microbiota is formed by microbes such as archaea protozoa, viruses, fungi, and, most of all, our friends, bacteria. The unicellular fungi are a lot larger than the bacteria, and their role is to clean up the gastrointestinal tract (gut) by mopping up junk and undigested food scraps. However, if you start to feed the fungi with junk such as sugar, they can turn aggressive and harm you—this is why it is very important to look after your microbiota. The collective genes of the microbiota are known as a microbiome. Mapping the microbiome is what has driven the current microbiotic revolution forward. Microbes live everywhere on and inside your body, but nearly all microbiota—99 percent—are found in the gut. And of all the microbes in the gut, 90 percent are bacteria rather than archaea, protozoa, etc. This is why the term *microbiota* can be used synonymously with gut flora. From now on, I will use the terms gut bacteria and gut flora instead of microbes and *microbiota*.

## Hardworking and multitalented

Apart from the fact that bacteria created all life on earth, they also continue to be essential to our world. For example, they cleanse poisons and toxins from our body. And did you know that photosynthetic bacteria in the sea create half of the oxygen we take in with every breath, as well as bind an equal amount of carbon dioxide? Bacteria are such an essential part of our lives that we have even outsourced some of our most important bodily functions to them—they digest our food, create vitamins and minerals, protect us from disease, and strengthen our immune system. They even produce substances that affect the way we smell—including our less palatable odors. They release signals that promote growth in our bodies and influence the development of our nervous system, mood, behavior, and the list goes on. Despite the fact that bacteria are tiny and invisible to the naked eye, while lacking a brain and a nucleus (unlike us), they still beat us by a mile when it comes to being multitalented. They also have an impressive ability to adapt to extreme environments. So the next time you have an irritating infection, think about all the fantastic things bacteria do for us. Bacteria are without a doubt evolution's geniuses.

**Some examples of essential tasks we have outsourced to our gut bacteria**

- They break down food we can't eat
- They break down carbohydrates, protein, and fat
- They produce vitamins
- They strengthen our immune system
- They convert hormones
- They provide our gut with energy
- They can detoxify painkillers
- They produce acids and gases

# *Bacteria's bad reputation*

In light of the fact that bacteria are the origin of all life forms, they are the reason I'm writing this book and you're reading it at this exact point in time. If this is the case, one might wonder why evolution's virtuosos have gotten such a bad reputation!

## Fear pays!

For a long time, bacteria have had a bad reputation among humans. Even in this day and age, most of us see bacteria as unwelcome disease carriers that we have to avoid at all costs. It's not surprising if you think about it. Traumatic epidemics such as the plague killed almost half of Europe's population during the fourteenth century, when 200 million people died. Other diseases have also left deep cultural scars in our memories. Even in modern times, the media have jumped on the bandwagon, giving us one terrifying story after another. When everyday items such as keyboards and cell phones are shown to be teeming with more "disgusting" bacteria than a lavatory seat, the media go into overdrive and happily reap the rewards of their magazines flying off the shelves. The basic message has always been that all bacteria are dirty, dangerous, and nasty carriers of disease. Unsurprisingly, some people have a phobia of bacteria. However, this one-sided view is deeply twisted, unfair, and simply wrong. The fact is that less than one hundred species of bacteria cause infectious diseases in humans, while thousands of other species are harmless and even essential for our body to function. Sadly, the media is rarely interested in giving a balanced view of reality.

It is not just the media that have given bacteria such an undeserved reputation. Their bad image might also be caused by the fact that they are invisible to the naked eye, and thus we usually only notice the negative consequences of bacteria. Who hasn't sneezed loudly during a quiet church service, suffered an incredible earache from an abscessed ear infection that refuses to go, or had an awful stomach upset with painful cramps? Most of us only notice bacteria when they make us ill, so it is not so strange that most of us view them as the bad guys.

## Without bacteria, society collapses!

Researchers have simply not had the right tools to dissect the world of bacteria—until now. It has only been recently that scientists have realized how important bacteria are to our health. The evidence is so overwhelming these days that scientists agree that bacteria's bad reputation is completely undeserved, something this book is trying to prove. Deep-seated truths have a tendency to stick, so let's conduct a thought experiment so you can see your bacteria in a new light: imagine what scientists believe would happen if all bacteria suddenly disappeared from the surface of the earth. Sure, it would mean that certain infections would be a mere memory, but at the same time it also means most plants and animals would die, resulting in a total breakdown of the food chain and therefore a huge reduction in our population. Without bacteria, society would collapse within a year. For too long, we have ignored and feared these very important bacteria, and it is time we start to appreciate them. If we don't, our understanding of ourselves, our origins, and our future health will be hugely deprived.

## *The discovery of a new organ*

For a long time, researchers viewed our intestines as long, sloppy, fleshy tubes whose job was to digest the food we ate and push undigested scraps through in the form of feces. The large intestine was seen as a fat sausage that absorbed water and salt and got rid of gas and waste, which was not very impressive from a biological perspective and, as it turned out, an incorrect assumption. With the discovery of gut flora, that is, the bacteria in our gastrointestinal tract, and its increasing amount of intelligent functions, our attitude toward it is very different today.

Researchers around the world suggest that we can no longer discuss our health without describing the central functions that bacteria have. They have even agreed that gut flora fulfill the criteria of an organ.

These days, gut flora, together with our gut, are known as our new "super organ." Let's take a closer look at it.

### Our new super organ

Thanks to new research, a new super organ has been "discovered" in our bodies well into the twenty-first century. We have known of the existence of the gut and gut flora but have been unaware of their central role to our brain function and mental health until now. Our gut flora weighs around the same as our brain or liver, about two to four pounds. And speaking of the liver, gut flora has a metabolic rate that surpasses the liver a hundred times over. In addition, 90 percent of all serotonin, which is a neurotransmitter that affects your mood and can lead to depression if there is an imbalance, is created in the gut. As if this wasn't enough, 80 percent of your immune system's cells can be found in the gut. The gut is therefore the largest immunological organ in our body, and so it's not surprising that more people are calling the gut and gut flora our new super organ. The brain and heart need to watch out—they have some serious competition!

### A pioneer without modern technology

How is it possible that it's taken humans so long—up until the twenty-first century—to discover a new organ? The answer is inadequate microscopes. It's a bit like Christopher Columbus missing the discovery of a new continent due to bad binoculars. Legendary scientists such as Charles Darwin have been accused of only focusing on large multicellular life-forms that can be seen with the naked eye and that live on the earth's surface. But Darwin actually did collect bacteria; however, the limitations of technology meant that he could not continue his research. The honor of discovering bacteria is actually bestowed on a Dutch man, Antonie van Leeuwenhoek. With the help of a homemade microscope, he saw bacteria in a drop of rain in the year 1674, and since then technology has developed at a huge pace.

### A quick journey through the gut

Maybe you consider the gut to be a long, sloppy thing that you never see, but in reality you look into it twice a day when you brush your teeth—the mouth is actually the entrance to your gut. This is where digestion begins with the help of your jaw muscles chewing—your body's own super blender. The masticated food passes to the long small intestine with its creases that actively and elegantly pump the food forward. The food substance then moves into the large intestine where most of the gut bacteria reside.

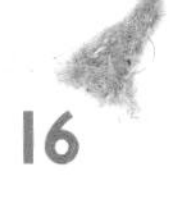



### Feces beats the iPhone in data capacity

From the first bite at the entrance of the gut (the mouth) to the last gut stop (the rectum), it takes roughly twenty-four hours before poo lands in the toilet. A healthy metabolism means that the gut empties at least once a day, with the feces being medium-soft and not hard. It should basically be a simple and fairly odorless process to empty your gut.

Inside the mouth you will find only a hundred bacteria per milliliter of saliva. In the upper part of the small intestine there are also relatively few bacteria as stomach acid and bile, which is extremely antibacterial, kill them off before they reach the intestine. Levels of bacteria in the small intestine then gradually rise again and max out in the large intestine. The main rule is that the nearer you are to the last stop in the gut, the more gut bacteria there will be; in fact, more than half of your poo is made up of bacteria, and in a gram of poo you will find 100 billion bacteria—that's fourteen times the human population on earth! If we were to look at the memory capacity that the genetic information in a gram of poo contains, it's the equivalent of 100,000,000,000,000,000 bytes—which is equivalent to over 93 million gigabytes. And here I was thinking that my iPhone had a lot of memory! By the way, did you know that every time you go to the toilet to empty your bowels, you empty the large intestine of a third of all its gut bacteria? But don't worry, the bacteria will regenerate in a day.

## *A closer look at gut bacteria*

The macrobiotic world is magical and full of life that is working hard twenty-four hours a day to keep you happy and healthy. Bacteria are so tiny that a million of them could dance on the head of a pin. Despite having trillions of these little guys in your gut, you will never see these colorful organisms (unless you have access to an advanced microscope); most of us will only ever notice the tangible consequences of these bacteria. So to give you an idea of the trillions of bacteria in your body, it is time to take a closer look at gut flora.

### As many bacteria as human cells

Bacteria truly are everywhere. A study conducted in 1972 and often quoted in the media suggests that there are 100 trillion bacteria and 10 trillion cells in an adult human body. This has resulted in the myth of 10:1, which suggests that we consist of ten times more bacteria than human cells. Many have even jokingly suggested that humans should be redefined as a bacterial colony. However, the latest figures estimate that humans have 39 trillion bacteria and 30 trillion human cells, so the ratio is more of 1:1. Regardless of the exact figure, that's a lot of bacteria—more than the number of stars in our galaxy (around 10 trillion). Each bacterium also has several thousand genes. That means that a human carries 100 to 150 times more genes from bacteria than they do from their own mother and father. Genetically speaking, you can say, albeit facetiously, that we are made up of 99 percent bacteria and 1 percent human.

### Different bacteria like different body parts

To construct the human bacterial map is a mammoth task that began in 2008 and is far from complete. However, so far it's been found that every body part has its own special local bacterial fauna. For example, our skin is colonized by propionibacterium, corynebacterium, and staphylococcus, while the vagina mostly contains lactobacillus. Some bacteria prefer the



**Soki Choi reflects on ever-changing research and new definitions**

The research connecting gut bacteria and the brain is evidently a new and changing field of study. Competing terms are everywhere and many people are trying to get their terms established. Shall we call it gut-brain axis, *microbiota-gut-brain axis*, or *mind-gut connection*? How do we define "psychobiotics" (see p. 90)? Should only probiotic bacteria be included or even prebiotic fiber? Discussions are firing up as a torrent of groundbreaking discoveries are being published.

**Soki Choi reflects on the gut's rise in stature from tube to brain**

Isn't it crazy that we have been carrying an organ as heavy as the brain for all these years and not known about it until now? Although we can't be sure, scientists believe that gut flora is the last human organ to be discovered! The gut and gut flora have gone from being considered waste-producing tubes lacking intelligence to being called our second brain. That is not a bad rise in status in a very short amount of time. Congratulations!



small intestine, others prefer the large intestine. The large intestine is full of bacteroides and bifidobacterium while the small intestine is dominated by lactobacillus and streptococcus. You can also find well-known bacterial species in the strangest of places, for example when a Japanese algae bacteria was found in the naval flora of a person who had never been to Japan. Did you know that only a sixth of the bacterial types on your right hand can be found on your left one? Or that the bacteria in your armpit has more in common with someone else's armpit than your own mouth? Different bacteria just like to inhabit different body parts.

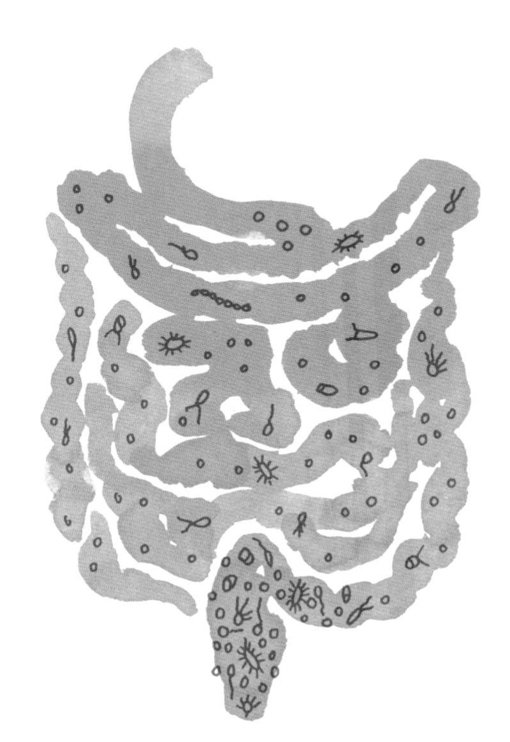

### Four main bacterial types in the gut

There's an infinite number of bacteria in your gut, especially in the large intestine. The gut flora is dominated by the four large bacterial phyla: Bacteroidetes, Firmicutes, Actinobacteria, and Proteobacteria. Of these, Bacteroidetes and Firmicutes are considered so important as an indicator of a healthy or sick gut that they form the basis of a popular gut flora index, the F/B ratio, which is like the BMI of gut flora. For example, overweight people have been shown to have a higher F/B ratio than slim people.

The gut flora is like a huge universe where new bacteria are constantly discovered. Currently researchers believe there are around one thousand different species in our gut with most bacteria (99 percent) belonging to around forty different species. The different species have long, elegant-sounding Latin names such as *Lactobacillus acidophilus* and *Bacteroides uniformis*. The species then divide into strains, such as *Lactobacillus acidophilus* LA-5. Within each strain, bacteria tend to be fairly similar; they eat the same food, have similar friends, and have similar abilities and properties. However, the reality is also not that simple. For example, *E. coli* is usually safe and even good for us, but the nasty variant EHEC can cause violent diarrhea and serious bleeds. Just remember that most bacteria are safe and helpful.

### You have a unique microbe signature

Each person has their own unique collection of bacteria on and inside their body, a bit like a bacterial fingerprint. This means that everything you touch (keyboard, cell phone, keys) contains your unique microbe signature. In addition, this unique microbe signature explains why a person with an excess of Firmicutes (see p. 20) can easily gain more weight even if eating exactly the same thing as their identical twin, while a person with an excess of christensenella (see p. 20) can eat as much chocolate cake as they like without gaining any weight. Unfair but true!

Having different gut flora also explains why one person can handle a moldy sandwich when someone else can't, or why acetaminophen can be more damaging to some people compared to others who may have gut bacteria that have the ability to detoxify this painkiller. Some people might also have stronger nerves than others if they have a large number of gut bacteria that produces lots of vitamin B, which is vital for our nervous system. All this makes the microbiotic world so exciting for researchers—it's not set in stone like our genes; instead it allows you to "manipulate" your gut flora to better your health. It's not surprising that many scientists are currently on the lookout to match specific bacteria with certain illnesses and health benefits.

In chapter 4 (p. 78), you will read more about how to strengthen your brain with the help of bacteria.

### Seven common gut bacteria

Before I start explaining what your gut bacteria can do for your health—and brain—let's look at the most common bacteria around. We have already established that bacteria are evolution's virtuosos. Our gut flora is like an orchestra that produces harmonies, in constant contact with other organs. When everything works smoothly, the body's instruments play in unison to create beautiful music of health and happiness. However, if the gut flora is not working as it should, the other instruments get confused and the musical arrangement that is our health suffers. Our little friends complete such advanced biochemical tasks twenty-four hours a day to keep us alive, and the only thing we have to do is give them some leftovers to eat and a place to stay in our gut.

It's now time to get to know some of the more common gut bacteria. No one is more important or better than the other; variety is the key to a potent gut flora.

#### BACTEROIDETES

Bacteroidetes is the most common bacterial type in our large intestine. The rod-shaped bacteria break down carbohydrates from plants as well as protein from animals. Those who eat more meat and fat have a lot of Bacteroidetes, which means Bacteroidetes are especially common in people with a Western diet. Bacteroidetes produce water-soluble vitamins such as B2, B5, B7, and C, which help them keep everything from colds to chapped lips at bay. In addition, they help keep away plant poisons from your gut. Bacteroidetes also create enzymes that can metabolize the burger and relish you have for lunch, or whatever else you might eat, acting a bit like beer when they convert sugar to yeast. The only drawback is that they can create some uncomfortable gases along the way.

#### FIRMICUTES

The specialty of Firmicutes is to digest, absorb, and store fat and sugar. People who have a lot of this bacteria prefer sweet and fatty foods, which is why it appears in abundance in overweight people and those who eat a Western diet. The ability of Firmicutes to store energy in fat cells was a huge advantage for the survival of humans hundreds of thousands of years ago, but today it means we sometimes eat too much and store excess fat. Overweight people generally have more Firmicutes and less Bacteroidetes, while healthier people tend to have more Bacteroidetes and less Firmicutes. In other words, it is worth aiming for as low an F/B ratio as possible for a healthy body.

#### CHRISTENSENELLA

*Christensenella* belongs to the phylum Firmicutes, but apart from that they are complete opposites from each other. This bacterial type is bad at extracting energy from food, which means people who have a lot of christensenella are slim and struggle to gain weight. They can eat a lot of chocolate, cake, and other sweet and fatty foods without putting on the pounds. Christensenella was discovered as late as 2011 and is still much of a mystery. Scientists believe that the existence of christensenella is genetic; however, this doesn't stop companies from selling expensive nutrients that they claim contain active christensenella.

#### *HELICOBACTER PYLORI*

*Helicobacter pylori* is 58,000 years old and appears in the stomachs in around half of the population. In 1982, the Australian doctor Barry Marshall discovered that most stomach ulcers were caused by this bacterial type, rather than stress or spicy food. With this discovery, Barry and his colleague were awarded the Nobel prize in 2005. Since then, stomach ulcers are treated with antibiotics. However, *H. pylori* is not all bad—it can also reduce indigestion and heartburn, thus reducing the risk of catarrh and cancer of the esophagus. Some scientists also believe that *H. pylori* can protect against asthma and allergies.

**PREVOTELLA**

Prevotella lives in the gut, mouth, and vagina. It was discovered by the French microbiologist André Romain Prévot in the 1920s. Prevotella breaks down the mucus that is produced by the gut. Its favorite food is vegetables with lots of fiber, which is why it is mainly found in large quantities in vegetarians. In a large study on children, scientists found no trace of prevotella in European children, but it was present in more than half the guts in African children. Prevotella produces B9 and B1, which is also known as thiamine (sulfur). Too little thiamine can lead to concentration problems, headaches, irritable moods, muscle shakes, and heart problems. The only drawback of prevotella is that is excretes unpleasant, sulfuric odors.



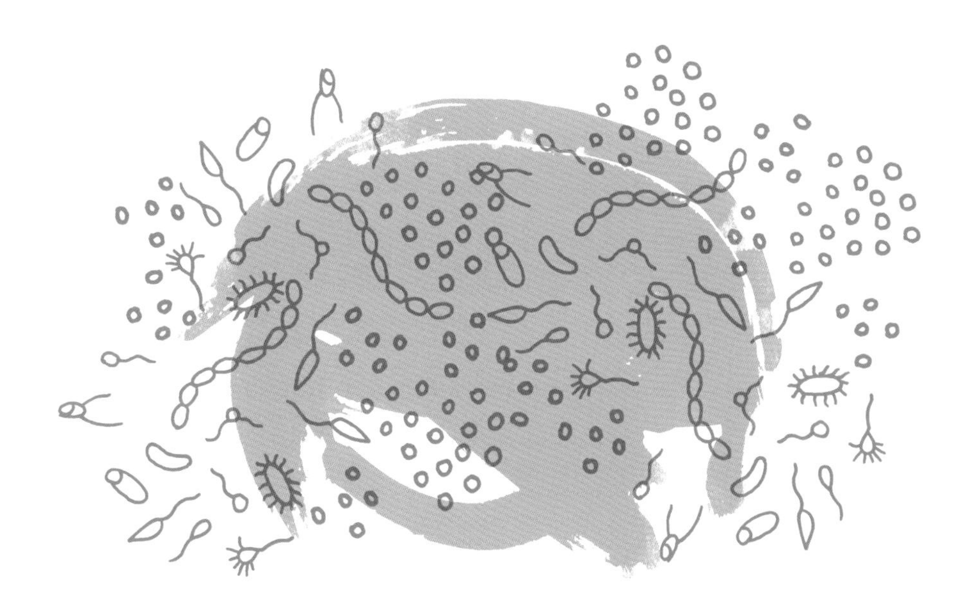

There are around one thousand different species of bacteria in our gut, but most of the bacteria belong to around forty species.

### BIFIDOBACTERIUM

*Bifidobacterium* is a common bacterial type that can be found in sour milk and yogurt, as well as breast milk. Different kinds of bifidobacterium have different properties. For example, *B. animalis* works against constipation, diarrhea, salmonella, eczema, and so on, while *B. longum* looks after our more complicated stomach problems such as ulcerative colitis and irritable bowel syndrome (IBS). A Swedish study also shows that *B. lactis* (together with *L. acidophilus*) can reduce inflammation and slow down the growth of cancer cells in the large intestine by stimulating the production of the anti-inflammatory butyric acid.

### LACTOBACILLUS

*Lactobacillus* is a well-known group of lactic acid bacteria that can be found in copious amounts in fermented foods such as yogurt, sauerkraut, kimchi, and kombucha. In the human body, this lactic acid bacteria occur mostly in the vagina (in women of European ancestry), and a lack of it can cause candida yeast in women. Apart from protecting you against nasty bacteria and yeast, lactobacilli also plays a part in stimulating the production of immune cells that protect you against infections, prevent diarrhea, reduce bad cholesterol and weight gain, and prevent allergies and eczema.

## Sky-high expectations from our gut bacteria

In order to learn about the bacteria on and in human bodies, scientists enthusiastically apply cotton buds all over our bodies to get samples. Bacteria and other germs on the skin can easily be removed from the body and studied in a lab. However, it's not always that easy to get to know our gut bacteria,. which are fussy and particular about the environment they can thrive in. They enjoy our moist, protective gut, where they are constantly fed with digested food.

This is the reason gut bacteria do not survive outside the body. If you remove bacteria from the gut, they will simply die. So, despite the huge promise and expectations in studying gut bacteria, the process takes a lot of work. We can study specific genes if we know what we are looking for—for example, scientists can show that infants have more active genes that break down breast milk than adults and that this bacteria later disappear with age. This is a viable study to conduct with a fairly obvious hypothesis, as adults don't need help breaking down breast milk. But at this moment, we don't have an overarching view of all our gut bacteria genes at the same time. And yet, even though research is in its infancy, the amount of published articles around the topic is increasing rapidly. Huge research projects—such as the American Gut Project and the British Gut Project—have commenced with aspirational goals. After spending several hundred years on the periphery of science, gut bacteria are now firmly in the center.

### Gut flora and your health

- The gut contains good bacteria that feed on fiber from vegetables and fruit. There are even bad bacteria that feed off stress and foods with lots of sugar and unhealthy fats.
- Having many different bacterial species is a sign of a healthy gut flora, therefore it's good to eat a variety of foods and avoid antibiotics (as antibiotics eliminate bacteria).
- A healthy gut flora with lots of different bacterial species strengthens your immune system and protects you against a host of chronic modern diseases and mental health issues.
- People with autism, ADHD, depression, anxiety, Alzheimer's, and Parkinson's share the common fact that their gut flora seems to have less diversity and larger numbers of bad bacteria than healthy people do (see chapter 3).
- Fibrous and fermented foods can protect your brain against mental health disorders. Fermented food can be found in yogurt, kimchi, and kombucha among other things.

# *Gut bacteria, inflammation, and the immune system*

Bacteria have many functions that are important to our health. Not only do they produce essential vitamins and other nutrients, they also help to convert several of our most important hormones. In recent years it's been discovered that gut bacteria also affect the brain through our immune system. Among other things, researchers have discovered a direct entrance to the brain through the so-called lymphatic capillaries, which could be an important link between the brain and gut flora. Before we look closer at how gut bacteria impacts the brain through our immune system, it is important to have a basic understanding of how the immune system works. This chapter will provide a beginner's guide to some of the basic aspects of the immune system, starting with an explanation of what inflammation is.

## The basics of inflammation

Your immune system consists of a complex network of cells, tissue, and organs that work together to protect you from bacteria and viruses that can cause illness. When you're infected by these foreign bodies, your body automatically creates inflammation to remove any disturbances and begin the healing of damaged tissue. Usually the infection starts the inflammation, but inflammation can also be triggered by other injuries such as physical trauma, heat, cold, and substances that induce allergies. Essentially, inflammation is the body's reaction to an injury.

### ACUTE INFLAMMATION IS GOOD

If you have a viral infection, inflammation will begin by localizing and removing the damaging substance that has caused the infection. The immune system activates and the affected cells release chemical substances that cause blood vessels in the vicinity to expand. Blood flow increases to the damaged skin or tissue, which becomes swollen, warm, and red due to the fluid that collects. Simply speaking, inflammation aids the body in looking after injuries—in other words, inflammation is good, even if the concept is usually associated with something negative. Acute inflammation also passes fairly quickly. The problem only begins when inflammation lasts too long, which can have devastating consequences for your health.

#### CHRONIC INFLAMMATION IS BAD

An acute inflammation that doesn't get better by itself becomes a chronic inflammation, which means that the immune system locks down and starts to become confused and acts destructively. Chronic inflammation also appears in tissue and organs inside the body, which makes them hard to find. This means that many of us walk around with undetected low-level inflammation that is allowed to develop over several years to become more severe illnesses.

Since the word inflammation comes from the Latin word *inflammare*, which means "fire," let's use the fire department as a metaphor to better understand what happens in a chronic inflammation.

When an acute inflammation appears, the body's loyal firefighters come along with their sirens to take care of the virus. When the virus has been dealt with, it is time for the tired firemen (the immune cells) to retire and recover so they can be ready for the next fire (inflammation). In chronic inflammation, a low-level fire continues to burn constantly, which means that the tired firemen carry on working twenty-four hours a day with no rest. An overactive fire service (the immune system) ends up so exhausted from lack of sleep that the firemen (the immune cells) start to behave In a confused way, for example by burning their own tissue or attacking friendly bacteria.

#### INFLAMED BRAIN

A tired and confused immune system turns "friends into enemies." This means that cells start to damage their own tissue instead of protecting it, which is what happens in autoimmune diseases such as multiple sclerosis (MS) and rheumatism. Some cells react so destructively from chronic inflammation that they even "commit suicide." This phenomenon is known as apoptosis and it hits our brain the hardest as the brain can't build new nerve cells as quickly as, say, a muscle can.

Chronic inflammation can also disturb nerve impulses so that messages from the brain don't reach other parts of the body, like the fingers. The results can be involuntary shaking or an inability to move the muscles, as happens in Parkinson's. Inflammation in the nervous system has recently become a hot topic within research, as inflammation in the brain has been shown to be connected to depression, Alzheimer's, and Parkinson's. In medical terms, a brain inflammation is now known as neuroinflammation, a term worth memorizing.

#### IS INFLAMMATION THE ROOT OF ALL ILLNESS?

Humans react differently to chronic inflammation. Asthma, for example, is usually an effect of long-term local inflammation in the lungs, while chronic inflammation in the muscles results in loss of muscle mass. Sneaky cancer tumors, on the other hand, use the immune system to hasten their own growth. Many conditions also connect in a vicious circle—for example, research shows that in obesity and chronic inflammation, the body's cells are in a heightened state of stress, which in turn activates chronic inflammation in the body's blood vessels. This leads to the narrowing of the arteries and arteriosclerosis, which then increases the risk for heart disease and premature death. If we remove heritability from the picture, many scientists and doctors suspect that many, if not all, chronic illnesses originate from chronic inflammation. Some of the illnesses that have been shown to have long-term inflammation at its core are allergies, Alzheimer's, asthma, arthritis, arteriosclerosis, cancer, Chron's disease, diabetes, heart disease, skin disorders such as psoriasis and eczema, IBS, MS, rheumatoid arthritis, and ulcerative colitis. That's why it's smart to keep an eye on the level of inflammation in your body.

#### WATCH OUT FOR CYTOKINES

If you haven't already heard about cytokines, it's something you need to keep an eye on in both an inflammatory and a microbiotic context. Cytokines are a deciding factor in several processes among the immune system, gut bacteria, and the brain.

Cytokines are the immune system's own neurotransmitters—our chemical messengers. This means that when your immune system sends signals to the brain, for example regarding an infection, it's the cytokines that carry the message. Cytokines regulate direct inflammation, healing, and other processes. When you are ill, cytokines make you feel sick (fever, feeling tired, aches, etc.), and when you take medicine to reduce your temperature, it is the cytokines that are inhibited. Cytokines, which consist of proteins, are produced by special immune cells when needed. There are around 150 different types of cytokines, some of which promote inflammation and others of which reduce inflammation. This means that there are both good and bad cytokines.

### Your immune system is in your gut

What does your immune system have to do with your gut? Well, 80 percent of the immune system's cells are in the intestinal tract, which makes the gut the largest immunological organ in the body. Apart from allowing nutrients into the blood, the gut stops toxins and foreign bodies from making us ill. If the balance between good and bad bacteria is disturbed, the immune system reacts immediately.

#### MICROBIOTIC BOOT CAMP

In the gut, there are cavities where your immune cells can play with your gut bacteria safely and without distraction, and without causing danger to your body. It is like a microbiotic boot camp where the immune cells learn to differentiate between foreign bacteria and human body cells, among other things. But this exercise can prove challenging because outwardly, bacteria can look like human cells, and therefore a confused immune system can start to attack the body's own tissue if they mistakenly believe that it is bad bacteria. This happens in the cases of autoimmune diseases such as MS and rheumatism.

Another reason for this boot camp is that immune cells need to learn to control their innate defense mechanisms so they don't automatically target all bacteria. By practicing differentiating between good and bad bacteria, the trained immune cells will learn to react wisely when they meet different types of bacteria. Fully trained immune cells are constantly sensing all the bacteria that passes in the gut, and as soon as they discover unwanted intruders, they start up the immune system to reduce the harm.

Bad bacteria like to hide in the intestinal villus. But in a healthy body, whenever bad bacteria try and settle down in the intestine, we can thank the good gut bacteria as they will have already gotten there and taken all the good spots. This is known as colonization, and it is the typical way in which good bacteria protect you against disease-causing bacteria. Peaceful species of bacteria have also been shown to make the immune system less aggressive by stimulating the production of more friendly immune cells.

#### WATCH OUT FOR "FIREBOMB" BACTERIA!

Out in the real world, immune cells will stumble upon both good and bad bacteria. There is a particularly nasty group of bacteria that are equipped with a strong poison, which acts as a firebomb that ignites the process of inflammations, hence the name. These damaging firebomb bacteria can be found in copious amounts in people who eat a typically Western diet with a high amount of animal fat and sugar.

The chemical name of the firebomb compound is LPS (lipopolysaccharide), and it consists of a nasty mix of fat (lipids) and sugar (saccharide). The main task of LPS is to protect and give solidity and structure to the firebomb bacteria's cell walls, and so long as the bacteria remain in the gut, all is fine. The problem occurs when large amounts of firebomb bacteria die, which they frequently do, and large amounts of LPS are released straight into the bloodstream, which quickly trigger strong inflammations. In addition, LPS loosen the gut barrier, resulting in even more of this bacterial toxin seeping through the barrier and worsening an existing inflammation in a vicious circle. The levels of LPS in the blood is therefore a good indicator of the general level of inflammation, as well as the level of leakage in the gut.

Of all the problems caused by LPS, animal studies indicate learning difficulties and memory problems, which is why it is probably no coincidence that levels of LPS in people with Alzheimer's have been shown to be three times higher than in others. Elevated levels of LPS have also been found in people with depression, Parkinson's, and the deadly amyotrophic lateral sclerosis (ALS); and this list seems to increase daily. Researchers have noted that, among other things, LPS reduces the production of the protein BDNF, which is important for the creation of new brain cells and memory. BDNF also protects the brain against free radicals, toxic materials, and brain damage. That's all the more reason to immediately try to reduce the number of dangerous firebomb bacteria and increase the amount of good lactic acid bacteria in our guts. The easiest way to do this is to avoid junk food and eat fiber-rich and fermented foods, which you can find in kimchi and kombucha, among other things (see p. 111 for a full list).

# *Gut flora—from the cradle to the grave*

Over the course of life, your gut flora changes from the cradle to the grave. Generally, the number of bacterial species increases at the start of life and reduces toward the end of life. In between this, your gut flora's exact constitution depends on a range of lifestyle factors, such as where you live and what you eat. Research shows that how your gut flora is programmed and how it develops begins before you are even born. Previously, researchers thought that the uterus was sterile, but new studies show that there are traces of bacteria in the uterus. In other words, the mother's bacteria can be important to the child's health even before birth.

## How birth affects your gut flora

Before birth, children have no gut flora, which means that the child has not had a chance to train its immune system with its bacterial sparring partners. Babies born vaginally are covered in a myriad of good bacteria all at once, and research shows that birth is a deciding factor in setting up children's immune systems "correctly" for the development of a healthy gut flora and brain. In contrast, research shows that the bad bacteria a child's immune system first comes into contact with can contribute to them developing asthma, allergies, autism, anxiety, etc. Children born by cesarean section may encounter bad bacteria that is present on the mother or a doctor's skin and may even come into contact with harmful bacteria in the hospital environment (staff, equipment).

The fact that pregnant women have an abundance of beneficial lactic acid bacteria in the birth canal is probably evolution's way of giving children the absolute best start in life.

## A fully developed gut flora at ages two to three

The next important phase in the colonization of gut flora occurs through breastfeeding. Breast milk contains both probiotic bacteria and prebiotic fiber, therefore acting as a fertilizer to the child's bacterial garden. After around six months, even more bacteria appear in the breast milk, which work to break down carbohydrates—probably to prepare the child for solid foods. After this, the child's gut flora is shaped by everything they encounter in their environment, such as wet kisses and hugs from their nearest and dearest, as well as pets, or objects they put in the mouths.

By two to three years of age, a child's gut flora is pretty much fully developed and "adult." This doesn't mean that the gut flora doesn't change; it stays dynamic. However, it is no longer age but rather lifestyle-related factors such as food, exercise, illness, stress levels, antibiotics, and medication that shape the gut flora from here on.

## Teenage gut flora in the danger zone

Teenagers go through big lifestyle and hormonal changes and need to pay extra attention to their gut flora. Apart from irritating acne and emotional instability that plague many teenagers, other factors like bad diet, stress, lack of sleep, and alcohol can lead to a drastically impoverished gut flora. This in turn can make teenage anxiety and depression worse. As a result, the teenage years seem to be a time when gut flora and mental health are really in the danger zone. Researchers suggest that engaging in all the right decisions and changes that lead to a healthier gut flora during teenage years is a good investment in the brain and mental health for the future.

Parents should therefore be extra careful and encourage fiber-rich and fermented foods above one-sided diets (especially junk food) in their teenagers. More on which foods strengthen the gut flora and brain can be found in chapters 4 and 5.

## Eating your way to a "younger" gut flora

Bacterial variety and the amount of beneficial Bifido bacteria generally reduce in people starting from around seventy years of age. Italian research has increasingly found that some older people, age seventy and above, who ate a Mediterranean diet rich in fiber and lactic acid bacteria had a "younger" and healthier gut flora similar to that of a twenty-year-old. A similar study from Ireland showed that older people who ate a typical Western diet (with lots of saturated fat and sugar) had an "older" and unhealthier gut flora, that is to say one with less diversity and higher levels of the bacterial genus Firmicutes. Research suggests that a Western diet has the same effect on gut flora as age does. The good news is that it is evidently never too late to rejuvenate your gut flora through fiber-rich and fermented foods, which will result in a strengthening of your immune system and an addition of healthy years to your life, and an elevation of your mood—all at the same time. In chapters 4 (p. 78) and 5 (p. 112), I will share with you my best tips on how to rejuvenate your gut flora with good food. There are simply many good reasons to look after your gut flora through lifestyle and diet.

# *A summary of chapter 1*

**Bacteria—first life on earth**

• Bacteria are all over the planet and on or inside your body.

• Bacteria produce half of the oxygen you take in with every breath.

• Most bacteria are harmless and essential for you.

• Without bacteria, society would collapse within a year.

**Microbiota (gut flora)—a living ecosystem**

• Gut flora consists of bacteria, archaea, protozoa, viruses, and fungi.

• There are 39 trillion living microbes in your gut, more than the number of human cells in the body.

• Each person has their own unique bacterial fingerprint.

• Four groups of bacteria dominate the gut.

**The gut—our immune system**

• The gut is our largest immunological organ (320–430 square feet)

• 80 percent of the immune system's cells are located in the gut.

• Gut bacteria train the immune system.

**The large intestine is the home of bacteria**

• 99 percent of human microbes are in the gut.

• 90 percent of the gut's microbes are made up of bacteria.

• Most gut bacteria are in the large intestine.

• The closer to the gut's "exit," the higher the concentration of bacteria.

• A gram of poo contains a larger "memory capacity" than an iPhone.

CHAPTER 2

# The dialogue between the gut and brain

# *The gut-brain axis*

Did you know that your gut talks to your brain? Twenty-four hours a day, the gut sends huge amounts of biochemical information to your brain. This newly discovered connection between gut and brain is now known as our biochemical supercomputer.

Communication between the gut and brain goes both ways and passes, among other things, through the vagus nerve, the body's own broadband connection (see p. 45). Even if the data goes both ways, the largest flow of traffic goes from the gut to the brain. The brain's activities are therefore very dependent on information from the gut, while the gut is able to handle its activities on its own, without much help from the brain.

## Your second brain

The gut's own nervous system is made up of fifty to a hundred million nerve cells, which is as many as can be found in the whole spinal cord. That is why the nervous system in the gut is often called the second brain. In medical terms it is known as the enteric nervous system or ENS. This second brain collects information from the gut and sends it to your primary brain. A long time ago, evolutionarily speaking, the brain actually developed from this second brain. There are therefore many similarities between the enteric nervous system and our central nervous system. In the gut, for example, you will find the same neurotransmitters that are in the brain, such as serotonin, acetylcholine, and dopamine. Despite this, the enteric nervous system is not seen as part of the central nervous system; rather, it is part of the peripheral nervous system. The enteric nervous system, together with the sympathetic and parasympathetic nervous system, also belong to the autonomic nervous system, which deals with nonconscious activities.

Digestion is the best example of how the gut's nervous system works independently. It is a biochemical ballet where your second brain, together with an arsenal of neurotransmitters, direct and steer the activities in the gut; from the mouth to the intestinal exit. It's a complicated process that you're rarely aware of, even though it takes place twenty-four seven. More than 90 percent of all the information that collects in your gut never reaches your consciousness; instead there is a quiet dialogue in the background between the gut and brain. You'll only notice your second brain when something is wrong, such as with food poisoning or an infection. In such cases, your second brain sends out nasty signals like stomachaches, heartburn, nausea, and vomiting. This also means that the primary brain inside your cranium will only take measures when you need to act, such as when it is time to start or stop eating or go to the toilet when you feel the effects of food poisoning.

If digestion and metabolism is the responsibility of your second brain, your primary brain has the overall responsibility for the body's condition as a whole. That's why your primary brain watches and collects information from several systems at the same time, with the gut's nervous system being one of them. This mass of information from all the organs, systems, and surrounding environment is constantly being integrated to achieve balance and equilibrium in the body.

### Your inner Big Brother

Your second brain, the gut's nervous system, is an advanced, sensitive, and high-achieving security system. It is comprised of a fishnet-like casing as large as a 430-square-foot apartment. This gigantic watchful net—your inner Big Brother—surrounds the esophagus, stomach, and intestinal walls. The net itself is made up of many sensory nerve cells that constantly watch and collect tons of biochemical data and information from all areas of the digestive system, whether it is tension in the gut, the composition of content of the gut, the level of acidity or water, and the amount of digestive hormones. The gut's nerve cells are very sensitive, which means you can have an overreaction toward certain foodstuffs, especially artificial additives that the gut doesn't recognize. That's why the nerve cells are protected on the inside of the intestinal wall so they can avoid coming into direct contact with food. The vulnerability of the gut's nerve cells also means that they can be damaged or die, which has been shown to create serious gut disruption associated with stomach and intestinal diseases such as IBS. Because of this, a hardier team of specially trained cells—endocrine cells and sensory neurons—work twenty-four seven to watch, register, and send, information regarding gut sensations to both your second brain and the primary brain.

To get a better understanding of your inner Big Brother, we will once again follow the food journey through the gastrointestinal tract. The journey begins in the palate, where taste receptors in the tongue sends signals to the rest of the gastrointestinal tract, which, strangely enough, also has taste receptors. Researchers believe that taste receptors in the gut don't have anything to do with taste in the mouth; rather, they send information to the brain, especially for "sweet" and "bitter" tastes. What is communicated in this gut-brain dialogue is not clear. When the food reaches the esophagus, the whole network of millions of sensors is activated in the whole gut and lights up like a watchful, flashing net. Along the whole gastrointestinal tract, every little activity of the food's journey is registered by the net and reported to its two "employers"—the second brain in your gut and the primary brain in your head who both tune in to the reports, but for different reasons.

Your second brain will want information from the gut primarily to optimize digestion. These digestion reports cover everything, from the size of the meal, chemical information regarding food content (fat, protein, carbohydrates), and concentration and consistency as well as the size of food particles. When your second brain receives information from the gut's Big Brother that you are eating food with, for example, a high fat content, it gives an order to the gut to slow down mechanical movements. For food with low calorific values, your second brain will tell the gut to increase the movements so that as many calories as possible can be absorbed. The digestive reports even include information about foreign bodies, such as dangerous bacteria, viruses, or other toxins in the food. If such a thing has entered the gastrointestinal system, your second brain makes sure that your gut takes in lots of water from the body and even changes direction of the gut's movements to flush the stranger out as quickly as possible through one or both of the gastrointestinal tract's exits.

Your second brain also works with the rest of the systems in the body, such as the hormonal system, which in medical terms is known as the endocrine system. Hormone-producing cells, or endocrine cells, are so numerous in the gut that if you were to press them together into a lump, it would without a doubt be the body's largest hormone-producing organ. When the endocrine cells send out hormones for hunger or fullness to your primary brain, this is when you become aware or conscious of your second brain.

For a long time, researchers were happy with the above description of the dialogue between the gut and brain; they believed it covered all aspects of the gut-brain connection. It therefore came as a total surprise when modern-day researchers after 2008 discovered trillions of lively bacteria chatting away in the gut, bacteria that not only took part in the gut-brain dialogue but that also played a role in the prevention and promotion of disease, both physical and psychological. We will now take a look at why bacteria are so important to our brain and mental health.

## *Gut bacteria are crucial for your brain*

Why are bacteria so important to our brain? It's not such a strange concept, really. Once again, all life—humans, Plants, and animals—comes from bacteria. The fact that we are defined by our bacteria is as obvious as the fact that we are defined by our genes; it has just taken humankind a bit longer to discover the bacterial world within us and its importance to our brain and mental health.

### Bacteria—your own mini-doctor

The reason our gut bacteria can affect and direct our behavior, mood, and mental health is partly because bacteria have a phenomenal ability to produce biochemical molecules that regulate our brain. In contrast to the short time pharmaceuticals and technical innovations have had to develop, these bacterial mini-doctors have had a long time to learn how to create signaling molecules—about three billion years. In a constant process of trial and error, trillions of mini-doctors have tirelessly developed and honed the signaling molecules that today fill our body's biochemical treasure chest with hormones, cytokines, peptides, neurotransmitters, etc. Throughout the years, our very own bacterial pharmaceutical factory in our gut has developed into a highly sophisticated, complex, and sensitive machine that, unless handled with great care and respect, can lead to serious defects (illnesses), as you'll soon see.

### Intelligent bacteria move into the gut

If bacteria really were earth's first living organisms, which have since proved themselves essential to our health, you might wonder how they ended up in our gastrointestinal tract in the first place. Here is how it happened: over 500

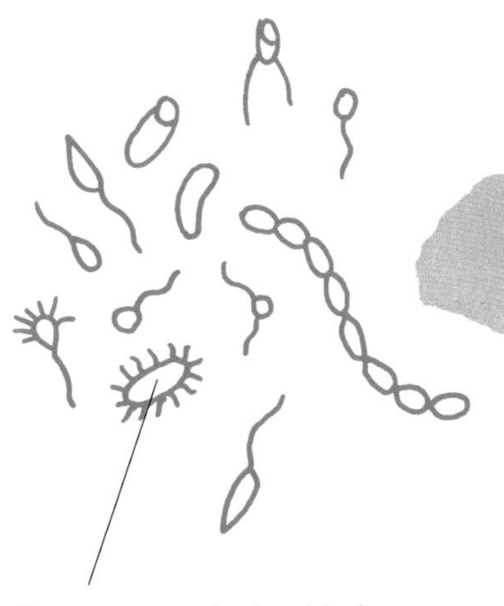

Bacteria were the first life-forms on earth.



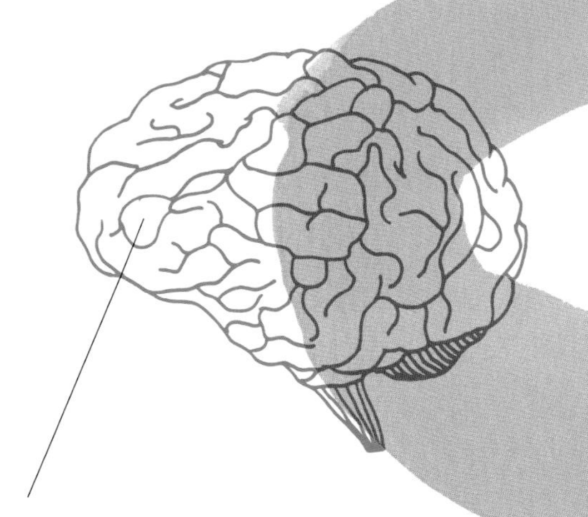

Our primary brain (the one inside the cranium) was born out of the gut's nervous system.

Today, bacteria, the gut, and the brain coexist and work together in the body.

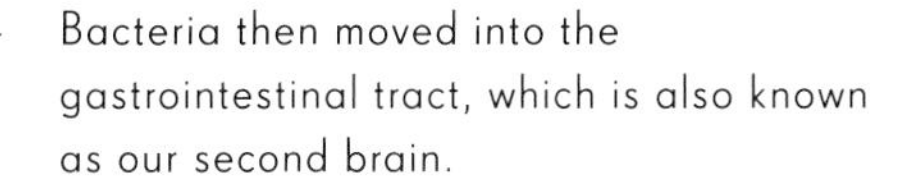

Bacteria then moved into the gastrointestinal tract, which is also known as our second brain.

million years ago (or 1.2 billion years, some say), the first multicellular organisms developed in the sea in the form of algae. Some bacteria came into contact with these tiny marine animals and eventually moved into their gastrointestinal system. This proved to be a good move that led to several benefits for both parties—the bacteria had a safe home where they could eat themselves full and get free transportation from place to place, while their marine hosts were aided in digestion, dealing with toxins, and benefiting from the many vitamins that their bacterial guests produced. Most of all, the marine hosts had access to these mini-doctors' recipes on different signaling molecules, recipes that had taken bacteria several billion years to develop.

## The gut—your own pharmaceutical factory

Once our bacterial mini-doctors moved into the gut, humans were given a shortcut and access to the enormous knowledge stored by bacteria on how to create valuable signaling molecules. The genetic intelligence from bacteria is what has made it possible for the nervous system in our gut to learn how to produce substances that guide our health, brain, and well-being today. For example, 90 percent of the body's serotonin is created in the gut and only 10 percent in the brain, and 50 percent of our reward chemical dopamine is produced in the gut. In other words, we have a whole pharmaceutical factory in our guts.

**Serotonin:**
A neurotransmitter that regulates worry, anxiety, sleep, wakefulness, pain, feelings of hunger and being full, etc. It even controls gut coordination.

**Dopamine:**
A neurotransmitter that is released in the brain when we experience a reward. It also controls fine motor movements.

**Noradrenaline:**
A neurotransmitter that, among other things, activates the body's fight-or-flight response. It is also important for our alertness.

## The brain was born from the gut's nervous system



Did you know that the gut's nervous system was the first nervous system to develop? As more complex organisms evolved, another nervous system grew from the gut's nervous system—the central nervous system. This new system was of course separate from the digestive system, but the two have always been closely connected. The central nervous system eventually established its headquarters at the top of the body, underneath the hard, protective cranium.

From the beginning, the gut's nervous system had responsibility for all behavior, including the ability to approach or retreat from another animal. This function was eventually outsourced to the limbic system, which is the part of the brain that regulates emotion. Along with the development of the central nervous system, the brain took on more responsibilities from the gut's nervous system. Finally, the brain inside the cranium was responsible for everything related to the outer world except digestion. The fact that the brain was created from the gut's nervous system proves the extremely intimate connection that exists between the gut and the brain.

## Your brain is formed by bacteria

There is no doubt that bacteria are required for the early development of the brain. During the first three years of life, a narrow window of opportunity also known as the neurodevelopmental window, colonization has to happen in order for our stress response system, the hypothalamic pituitary adrenal (HPA axis), and other parts of the brain to form normally. This window is when the brain seems to develop a lifelong capacity to handle stress, as well as the creation of brain cells. Typically, it is also during this vulnerable time that the gut-brain axis can encounter bacterial offenses such as cesarean sections and antibiotics (see p. 71).

To examine how important bacteria are to the brain, researchers studied "bacteria-free" mice. In order to "cultivate" mice without bacteria, they were born through caesarean section, fed sterile food, and grown in a sterile lab. What did the mice free from bacteria teach us? Of all the strange defects, the following are worth mentioning: atrophied intestines without villus, enormous appendixes, and slow digestion. They also had a completely different brain architecture as opposed to their genetically identical twins who grew up in a "normal" environment filled with bacteria. For example, the amygdala (one of the emotional centers in our brain) was enlarged, which has been linked to autism and anxiety disorders. Even the number of strangely formed brain cells (thin and hard) was increased, and the turnover of stress hormones was higher when compared to their bacteria-exposed mouse friends. The mice free from bacteria also had other genes that were activated, compared to the control group. Even their immune systems were noticeably weaker with fewer immune cells. We can say without a doubt that the brain deforms without bacteria. Bacteria are simply necessary for the brain.

# *A lifelong symbiosis*

Did you know that you and your bacteria live in a lifelong relationship until death do you part, whether you like it or not? It is a binding biological contract that has benefited all parties involved for the past five hundred million years; I call that a lifelong marriage! It can be useful to know that there are three types of symbiotic relationships that you and your bacteria might find yourselves in:

1) Commensalism: one party benefits without harming the other.
2) Mutualism: both parties benefit from each other.
3) Parasitism: one party benefits from the relationship while the other is harmed.

Let us take a closer look at the relationship between humans and bacteria.

## A win-win relationship

For a long time, researchers saw our relationship to bacteria as mainly parasitic and, in a best-case scenario, commensal. This has since been shown to be wrong; there is a clear ecological win-win mechanism between humans and bacteria. Bacteria have a privileged life in our gut, which includes free lodging, constant food through our undigested scraps, a pleasant temperature, and an unlimited opportunity to spread genetic information. They even have free "Wi-fi" as they can dial into the vagus nerve, the body's own super broadband (see p. 45), to take part in the biochemical data traffic that is constantly being sent back and forth between the gut and brain.

In return, the bacteria use this biochemical information about you to keep an eye on your stress levels, your emotional state, whether you are sleeping or awake, etc. The information is then used to adapt the production of biochemical substances such as hormones, vitamins, neurotransmitters, and metabolites (see p. 43). The bacteria also render harmless foreign bodies and toxins. In scientific terms, friendly bacteria are called symbionts. All they are interested in is that their host—you—reach optimal health levels, as this means a continued privileged lifestyle for them. A classic win-win relationship, in other words.

## Parasites in waiting

There are also disease-causing bacteria, called pathogens, that live and sleep in your gut. A gut flora dominated by bad bacteria means it produces more toxins, stress hormones, and other dangerous substances that benefit these parasites at the cost of your health. If there are more friendly bacteria than harmful ones, you should be fine, but if you start to mistreat your bacteria with stress, antibiotics, medication, and junk food, it won't take long for the pathogens to come to life, grow, and become the dominant bacterial population in your gut flora. The clever pathogens have also been shown to have a sneaky ability to change friendly bacteria into dangerous and harmful ones.

### Our oldest contract is in danger

Luckily, gut bacteria prefer to live in harmony with their human host, where they mainly spend time digesting food, growing, and reproducing without disturbing us. The price of starting a war with their host usually outweighs any gains. The same principle drives our immune system, which prefers not to use its sophisticated weapons against beneficial bacteria (immune cells learn early on to differentiate between good and bad bacteria). Instead both parties focus on giving each other mutually beneficial services. However, more and more scientists worry that the rapid increase of modern disease and mental health problems today is a sign that our oldest and most successful win-win contract with our health-promoting bacteria is at risk.

In chapter 4, I'll reveal some of the most serious crimes humans have committed against our contract with bacteria. I'll also address how you can start to repair and try to reinstate the contract between your bacteria and brain by changing your food and other lifestyle choices—we can make a difference!

## *The gut, its bacteria, and your emotions*

While other organs in the body do express themselves in certain ways based on each emotion, there is no organ that is as closely related to our emotions as the gut. Expressions like "butterflies in my stomach" and "my gut says . . ." and "I don't give a shit" reveal what many of us already know—that feelings and the gastrointestinal system are closely linked. New groundbreaking research even shows that bacteria in your gut are affected by what you feel and think.

We will now take a closer look at how your gut, bacteria, and emotions are connected.

### The gut and your emotions

A fascinating example of the intimate relationship between the gut and brain is revealed by the fact that every emotion that appears in your brain corresponds to a mechanical "grimace" in your gut. It's just like the face—you can tell immediately if someone is angry because the face scrunches up, the eyes narrow, lips go white, and the jaw tightens. The same thing happens if someone is sad—the face then relaxes and the gaze is lowered; maybe even a tear appears. Reading someone else's emotional state via their facial expressions is a universal skill that nature has given humans. Each emotion is linked to a specific facial expression regardless of nationality, ethnicity, culture, language, and history. Most people know this truth, that feelings are reflected in our face, but not everyone knows that every emotion also has an equivalent expression in the gut. Now let's see

**Soki Choi reflects over who's in charge of who**

Several researchers believe bacteria in your gut can influence your food preferences. For example, they believe that a naughty "McDonald's" bacteria can get you to crave a burger, which then causes these bacteria to continue to flourish in your gut. It doesn't matter that you know intellectually that junk food is bad for you; the bacteria in the gut are larger in number and smarter. They will crush your willpower by manipulating your hunger and hormones in order to ensure their survival. Similarly, this means that if you start to feed your gut flora with good foods like kimchi, the good "kimchi" bacteria will flourish and finally create such a strong kimchi craving that you'll do anything to keep eating kimchi (I know!). With trillions of bacterial friends in your gut, you don't have to rely on yourself; just exercise a bit of your own willpower and feed the good bacteria until your army has grown so big that they will make you crave healthy food. I call that a win-win!



what happens simultaneously in the face and the gastrointestinal tract when you feel angry or sad.

When you feel mad, the brain sends out a unique combination of nerve signals to your facial muscles. This same "I feel angry" loop is also sent to the stomach and intestines simultaneously. If you had a mirror inside your stomach, you would see that the intestines would have contracted and the stomach would have hissed and spat out phlegm, hydrochloric acid, and other acidic juices, all while digestion slowed down. This is equivalent to the intestines' "angry face."

When you feel down, the brain sends out another melodic loop, the "I'm feeling sad" loop. The facial muscles relax, usually with the corners of the mouth turned down. At the same time, the gastrointestinal system hears the same loop and also relaxes. This is partly because the production of serotonin has reduced—apart from its antidepressant properties, serotonin also induces digestive reflexes. The relaxation of the intestine does not mean it's taking a rejuvenating nap; rather, the intestine is reducing its movements, which can lead to constipation and other digestive problems. That's why it's not so strange that depression and anxiety often go hand in hand with gastrointestinal problems.

So what we call a gut feeling is therefore not just a made-up phrase or our imagination but a direct reflection of our emotional state. As a famous American gut and brain researcher said, "Sadly, most patients don't know that their gastrointestinal problems are a direct reflection of their emotional state. And even sadder is the fact that their doctors don't know this, either."

### Bacteria and your emotions

Doctor and researcher Emran Mayer suggests in his book *A Mind-Gut Connection* that the brain's signaling of emotions instruct the gut bacteria to adjust their production of chemical substances according to the current emotional state. He believes a feeling that is triggered by a thought in the brain sends chemical instructions to bacteria via the gut's nervous system. According to Mayer, this instruction can be viewed as a recipe for a cocktail that the brain asks the bacteria to mix—a recipe whose ingredients depend on your emotional state.

If, for example, you are feeling stressed, stress hormones like noradrenaline have been shown to make gut bacteria more dangerous, according to Mayer. Noradrenaline can activate genes in pathogenic (disease-enhancing) bacteria, which makes them more aggressive and increases their chances of survival. Several laboratories have shown that these pathogens can cause serious gut infections, stomach ulcers, and life-threatening blood poisoning. Stress can even get some gut bacteria to transform the noradrenaline you already have in your gut to a stronger variant: adrenaline. Stress also reduces your beneficial bacteria.

This change in gut flora therefore changes critical signaling pathways to the brain, which in turn contributes to the development of stress-related illnesses, such as anxiety and depression. The sad thing is that even if you are exposed to stress for only a short period of time, it has been shown to shift the proportions of the largest bacterial strains in your gut in favor of more inferior ones.

So the next time you are about to entertain a thought that might make you feel angry or stressed, remember the chain reaction of contracted intestines, stomach acids, and aggressive bacteria releasing toxic stress hormones into your body.

Thanks to new research on bacteria, the link between the gut, bacteria, and your emotions has become clearer.

## *How your gut bacteria talk to your brain*

The common saying "all roads lead to Rome" accurately describes all the paths by which your gut bacteria can reach your brain (or your "Rome"). Researchers have just begun mapping this knotted labyrinth without maps and compasses, and it is easy to get lost in this newly discovered colossal world within us. Luckily, research has already revealed a few main clues, enabling us to discover the space between the gut and brain.

### Gut bacteria and neurotransmitters

A powerful way for gut bacteria to affect your brain is via neurotransmitters, of which a large amount is produced by gut bacteria. When gut bacteria consume indigestible food scraps (fiber), they spit out neurotransmitters as a by-product. So, what is a neurotransmitter? Neurotransmitters are the messengers of the brain that control our nervous system by turning the nerve cells on and off. Essentially, it goes like this: when nerve cell A wants to

THE CONVERSATION AMONG THE GUT, GUT BACTERIA, AND THE BRAIN

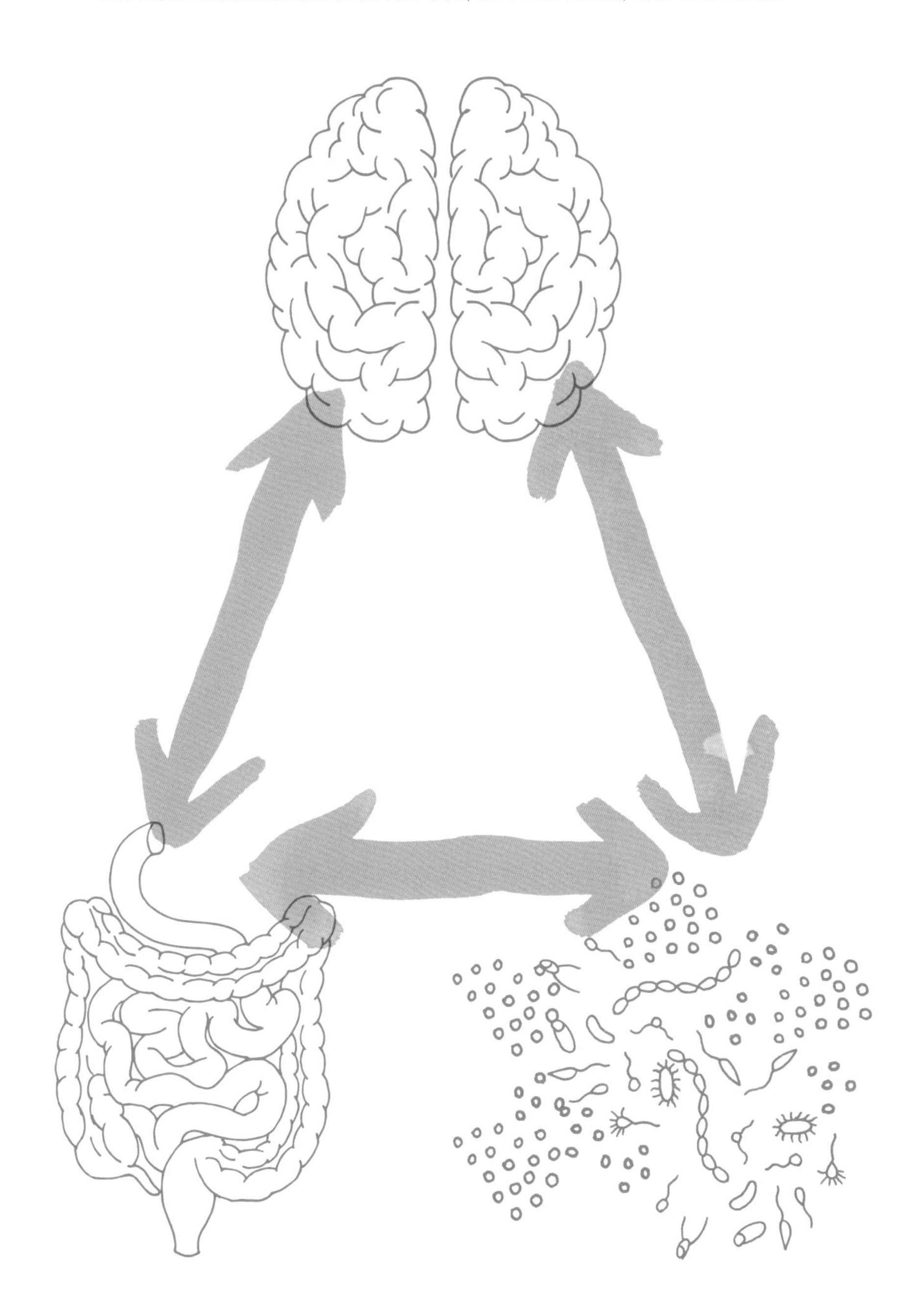

communicate with nerve cell B, nerve cell A releases a neurotransmitter that attaches to the receiving receptor of nerve cell B. So far, around fifty neurotransmitters have been mapped out, with the most common being serotonin, dopamine, adrenaline, noradrenaline, acetylcholine, and GABA. Neurotransmitters have to exist in the right amounts for us to feel well; too many or too few can cause various degrees of mental health problems. Out of everything that is controlled by neurotransmitters, here are a few worth mentioning: mood, wakefulness, sleep, sexual appetite, excitement, appetite, concentration, reward, motivation, memory, and movement. In other words, you and your brain are controlled by a chemical cocktail consisting of neurotransmitters. Apart from working with each other, neurotransmitters also interact with other cells, hormones, and genes in a complicated network that help to make you feel as healthy as possible.

The fact that we have a whole pharmaceutical factory in our gut that works twenty-four seven to change indigestible food scraps into neurotransmitters is a groundbreaking discovery.

As has already been mentioned, 90 percent of our happy molecule, serotonin, is produced in the gut and only 10 percent is produced in our brain. In addition, 50 percent of the reward molecule, dopamine, is produced in the gut, the same level as it is produced in the brain. Gut bacteria's mass production of neurotransmitters is a fundamental way in which bacteria can affect your brain and mental health.

#### SEROTONIN—THE ULTIMATE BRAIN-GUT SIGNAL

Serotonin is considered the ultimate neurotransmitter in the gut-brain axis as it is deeply integrated in both the gut and brain. You have probably heard that serotonin plays an important role in depression and is also known as the "feel good" or "happy" molecule. You are probably also aware that antidepressants, also called selective serotonin reuptake inhibitors (SSRIs), try to raise the serotonin levels in the brain. Lesser known is the fact that serotonin also plays an important role for gut movement, by contracting our intestinal muscles so that our foodstuffs are forcefully pushed forward. When you have acute food poisoning, serotonin's critical role in the gut becomes clear. The gut's nervous system gives an immediate order to evacuate the whole gastrointestinal system, and serotonin is released in large quantities. The increased concentration of serotonin creates nausea and speeds up gut movement to quickly remove the poisonous contents of the stomach. Here, serotonin shows off its unique ability to get the gut movement to change direction—in other words, to induce vomiting. Vomiting is so cleverly designed that just before the sour foodstuff flows out of our mouth, lots of saliva is produced to protect our teeth from corrosive stomach acids. So, too much of this "feel good" molecule can ironically make us feel awful, but all in the service of our health.

Now, over to the brain: when the amino acid tryptophan—the raw ingredient that produces serotonin—is ingested via food, it can be taken up by the blood and transported to the brain, where it is converted into serotonin, affecting your mood and mental well-being. Additionally, more and more researchers believe that the gut's enormous serotonin depot, which lies very close to the vagus nerve that connects the gut with the brain's emotional center, allows a constant stream of small doses of serotonin to reach the brain directly. It is possible that your nervous system and behavior adapt accordingly to this increased flow of serotonin to the brain via the vagus nerve; essentially, your gut bacteria can actually make you feel happier.

The dual role of serotonin in the brain and gut means that a serotonin level that is too low both lowers mood and slows down gut movement. This is why people who are depressed often have problems with constipation. Conversely, people with gastrointestinal problems (such as IBS) have been shown to have higher instances of depression, which is linked to a change in the gut's serotonin system. This two-way connection between the gut and brain shows that physical and psychological health are closely linked. The need to have an integrated and holistic approach within health care has never been clearer. More and more gastroenterologists (gut experts) and neurologists (brain experts) suggest that illnesses like depression and IBS could probably be clumped together as "gut-brain disease."

**How do you increase serotonin levels?**

Serotonin regulates worry, anxiety, sleep, wakefulness, pain, and even feelings of being full or hungry—yes, we have our happy molecule to thank for that feeling of satiation after a meal. Serotonin is extracted from the amino acid tryptophan, which the body gets through food since it can't produce it iself. Tryptophan can be found in protein-rich food (meat, fish, soya beans) and certain nuts and seeds (pumpkin and chia seeds). Access to tryptophan, and in turn serotonin, has been shown to depend on the presence of the lactic acid bacteria *Bifidobacterium infantis*. To maximize the body's serotonin levels, it is worth eating food rich in tryptophan and complementing that with lactic acid bacteria.

## Gut bacteria and metabolites

Another way for gut bacteria to affect the brain is through metabolites, which are the smallest particles that the body breaks food down into. Gut bacteria "chew" hard-to-digest fiber and then spit out various metabolites, such as bile, kaolin, and short-chain fatty acids. Short-chain fatty acids have especially been shown to have several positive effects on health. Let's take a closer look.

### SHORT-CHAIN FATTY ACIDS

In scientific terms, short-chain fatty acids are known as SCFA.

Short-chain fatty acids are one of the most important types of metabolites as they affect the nerve cells and work closely with our hormone system.

In simple terms, here is how it works: gut bacteria spit out short-chain fatty acids into the large intestine. Fatty acids speed up the release of hormone-producing cells in the gut. Then, together with these gut hormones, the fatty acids are released into the blood that reaches the brain, influencing our mental state. Besides fiber, the presence of lactic acid bacteria is also a good way to increase the production of short-chain fatty acids.

#### BUTYRIC ACID—THE STAR AMONG FATTY ACIDS

The big star among short-chain fatty acids is without a doubt butyric acid. It has been shown to have many positive effects, including having anti-inflammatory properties. In addition, butyric acid reduces the growth of bad bacteria, especially cancerous cells in the large intestines. Exciting research is currently being conducted on its effect on the brain and mental health, and it has even been linked to age-related illnesses, such as Alzheimer's and Parkinson's—for example, it increases the memory capacity in mice with Alzheimer's. Foods like kimchi and kombucha are the absolute best ways to get butyric acid in your system. Fiber that stimulates the production of butyric acid can also be found in foods with resistant starch, such as cold pasta, cold rice, cold potato, and potato flour (see more on p. 92).

> Butyric acid has been linked to age-related diseases, such as Alzheimer's and Parkinson's.

#### ACETATE—A ROGUE AMONG FATTY ACIDS

If there are stars, there are also rogues among short-chain fatty acids. Gut bacteria that produce the short-chain fatty acid acetate have been shown to control both our eating habits and how much weight we put on. This is because acetate can influence how much of the hunger hormone, ghrelin, and the satiety hormone, leptin, is released.

Acetate plays an important role in obesity. Gut bacteria produce acetate as a direct result of a fatty diet, so the consumption of more fatty foods will increase the amount of acetate, which increases the production of the hunger hormone, and so on. A vicious cycle is created, which in turn increases the risk of obesity and other health problems related to obesity. To break this cycle, you have to starve the acetate-producing bacteria and stop feeding them fatty foods—which is easier said than done.

### THE VAGUS NERVE—A CRITICAL LINK IN THE GUT-BRAIN AXIS

In order for substances produced by gut bacteria to reach the brain (neurotransmitters and metabolites), they have to choose from many routes. One obvious route is through the circulation of blood, and another central route is via the vagus nerve. The vagus nerve connects the gut to the brain, allowing for changes in the gut to nearly always be followed by changes in the brain, and vice versa. It's why psychological complications often follow digestive problems, as well as the other way around. The vagus nerve also regulates all aspects of the food's journey through the gut. If the vagus nerve only handled digestion and appetite, then its large amount of sensory fibers and the upward flow of information would not be needed. Above all, the vagus nerve acts mainly as a central signaling route between the gut bacteria and the brain.

**The vagus nerve—the body's own super broadband**

The vagus nerve is the longest of our nerves, going from the brainstem down to the gut. It actually consists of a pair of nerves that symmetrically weave their way down both sides of the spine. It is helpful to picture it as a thick cable, like the body's own super broadband. It consists of eighty thousand nerves that connect all of the body's organs (except the adrenal glands) to the brain. It spends 80 percent of its time collating data about what's going on in the body and 20 percent coordinating the body's unconscious activities. Mainly, it regulates the part of our autonomic nervous system that is activated at rest, that is, the parasympathetic nervous system. It can be anything from controlling the rhythm of your heart, digestion, gut movements, sweating, and the regulation of the pupils to urinating and sexual arousal. Since the vagus nerve has been shown to be sensitive to food, exercise, and stress, it is even more important to keep these lifestyle aspects in check.

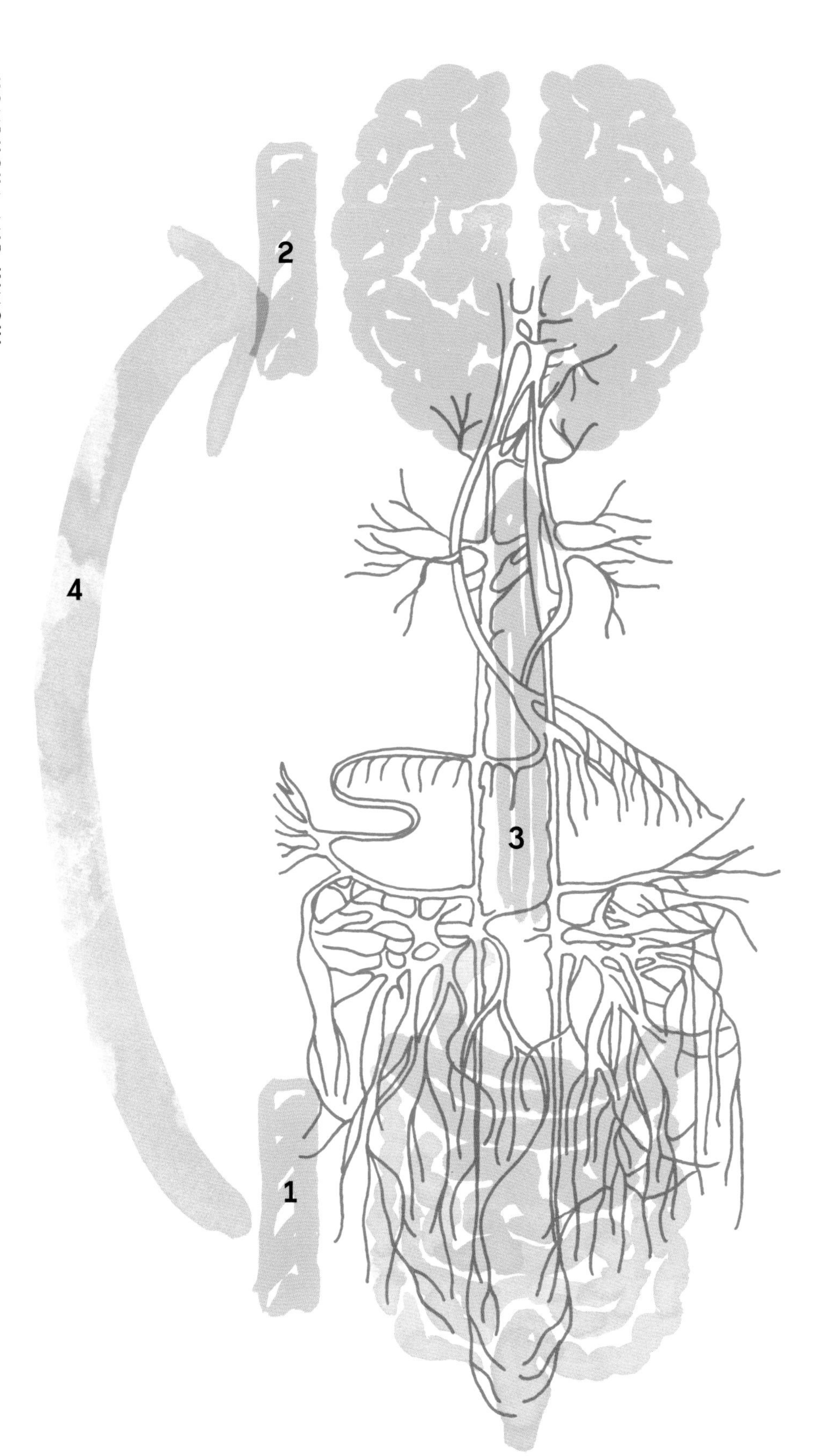
2
4
3
1

### The bacteria-brain map in a nutshell

**Two substances:** Gut bacteria produce two large groups of chemical messengers, neurotransmitters and metabolites, that affect your brain and your mental health. The neurotransmitter serotonin and the metabolite butyric acid are examples of beneficial substances produced by bacteria.

**Two barriers:** Gut bacteria's chemical messengers have to pass through two barriers to reach the brain: the gut barrier (1) and the blood-brain barrier (2). If the gut or blood-brain barriers leak and enable cytokines to inflame the brain, this can lead to depression and other brain-related diseases.
Two main routes: While many routes between the gut and brain exist, there are two main routes: the vagus nerve (3) and the blood (4). Even the immune system and the hormone system are involved, especially when bacteria use blood circulation to reach the brain.

**Two X-factors:** food and stress are two of the most decisive factors in the gut-brain axis. Chronic stress in combination with Westernized junk food drastically affect gut flora, which in turn can worsen mental health in a vicious circle.

**Two healing properties:** By feeding your gut flora with certain types of fiber, you stimulate bacteria's production of the anti-inflammatory butyric acid. Lactic acid bacteria reduces inflammation and heals a leaking gut or blood-brain barrier, and it can be found in fermented foods, such as kimchi and kombucha.

#### CUTTING THE VAGUS NERVE IS A BAD IDEA

Before doctors understood the pivotal role the vagus nerve plays, it was common to try and cure stomach ulcers by simply cutting the vagus nerve, also called a vagotomy. Even if this caused the production of stomach acids to stop, a host of unforeseen side effects appeared, such as heart palpitations, sweating, cramps, diarrhea, nausea, vomiting, and extreme fatigue. These days, vagotomies have been banned. Instead, new medical methods have been developed to stimulate the vagus nerve electronically to treat things like epilepsy, pain, and extreme depression where antidepressants have been ineffectual. New evidence has shown that both antidepressants and anti-anxiety medications affect the vagus nerve, suggesting that the vagus nerve might be a common route that these medicines take to reach the brain. As the vagus nerve is directly linked to the brain, stimulation of the vagus nerve is being investigated as a possible treatment for symptoms of autism and conditions like Alzheimer's.

## *The journey of bacteria through the immune system*

The immune system has been shown to play an important role in the dialogue between the gut and brain, especially when it comes to mental health. When bad bacteria come into contact with the gut's immune cells, the immune system immediately protects itself by producing cytokines (read more about these on p. 25). Cytokines enable the gut barrier to loosen up

**Soki Choi reflects on the health care of tomorrow**

We now know that the gut, brain, and gut bacteria communicate twenty-four seven and that any disruption in this communication can lead to chronic disease. In other words, it is clear that the gut and brain are intimately linked to each other. Despite this, traditional health care has partitioned our body and organized health care as if they were separate, unrelated parts of the body, such as ear, nose, and throat; head; or stomach. After having researched and worked for ten years within the health care industry, I can sadly confirm that researchers and doctors within various specialties don't usually communicate. Not only that, specialists within the same field also don't talk to each other. At the same time, groundbreaking research clearly points to the fact that it is necessary to view the human body as a holistic system, especially when it concerns the gut-brain axis. A health-care system that divides the body up into different parts invokes the idea of medieval practices.

In a world where we are used to updating the operating systems of our mobile phones at least once a week, it is rather incongruent that we find ourselves living with an extremely dated health-care system that does not reflect the complexities of the human body. Instead, the health-care system we have is one in which both doctor and patient can easily get lost in a dense jungle. Bearing in mind that health problems are escalating across the globe, it is only a matter of time before health care is forced to update its systems. How this might occur is hard to predict, but one thing is certain—our future health care needs to better reflect the intimate links among the body's different organs. I'm hoping the current research on the gut-brain axis can speed up the shift to a more modern system, dominated by an integrated and holistic perspective.

(leaky gut), which means harmful cytokines are released into the blood and inflame the body. The cytokines then reach the critical blood-brain barrier via the body's blood circulation, passing through to inflame the brain. In addition, more and more studies show that inflammation of the brain (neuroinflammation) is behind several of our most common brain-related diseases, such as depression and Alzheimer's.

### When the gut barrier leaks (leaky gut syndrome)

The gut barrier is made up of a tightly protective joint whose job is to prevent harmful bacteria, toxins, and other dangerous substances from being released into the bloodstream. Various factors like stress and junk food can make the gut barrier thinner, more porous, and prone to leaking. If your gut barrier becomes permeable and starts to leak, it sadly opens up the floodgates for disease-promoting bacteria and harmful substances to reach the blood and cause havoc. When a gut leaks, harmful bacteria start to move and come into direct contact with the gut's immune cells. The provoked immune cells don't like this, and they react in defense by spraying out cytokines that go straight into your bloodstream and infect your body and, in a worst case scenario, your mind. This is why you should keep your gut barrier leakproof—make sure to avoid chronic stress, which has been shown to loosen the gut's mucous membrane and increase the amount of harmful bacteria while also making them more aggressive (see p. 55), which in turn worsens ongoing inflammation and a leaky gut.

### When the blood-brain barrier leaks (blood-brain leakage)

Many of our chronic, first-world illnesses, such as diabetes and cancer, are believed to be caused by inflammation. For our most precious organ, the brain, to be inflamed, inflammation-enhancing substances like cytokines need to pass through the important blood-brain barrier. The blood-brain barrier consists of tightly forged walls of blood vessels that prevent harmful substances (infections, medications, drugs, microorganisms, and so on) from leaving their path and reaching the nerve cells in the brain and spine. The blood-brain barrier therefore protects the brain tissue, only allowing certain substances to pass through, such as oxygen, glucose, and amino acids. The rate at which things can pass through the barrier increase with brain damage (such as hemorrhages), heart attacks, meningitis, and even aging. Large leakages in the blood-brain barrier have also been found in people with dementia. In other words, the blood-brain barrier is a vital protection that simply must not leak.

Inflammatory substances like cytokines and lipopolysaccharide (LPS) have, in addition to their treacherous ability to loosen the gut barrier, been shown to loosen the vital blood-brain barrier, which allows them to reach the brain tissue and cause inflammation in the brain. Brain inflammation, or neuroinflammation, is frequently linked to some of our more common brain-related diseases, such as depression, anxiety, Alzheimer's, Parkinson's, and so on.

### Many harmful roads lead to "Rome"

Inflammatory substances can reach and affect the brain in a few other ways. Cytokines, for example, can affect communication in the brain by changing the concentration of neurotransmitters like serotonin, dopamine, and glutamine. Cytokines can also stimulate the release of other strong inflammation-enhancing substances (prostaglandins), which can make an existing inflammation worse. Recently, researchers have also discovered another way in which cytokines can directly affect the brain—by passing through the central lymphatic vessels in the lower side of the brain. There are many roads for inflammation-enhancing substances to reach "Rome," and one thing is for sure: inflammatory substances do not belong in our brain.



### Lactic acid bacteria repair gut and brain leakage

Researchers like to bring up inflammation-enhancing bacteria as soon as gut bacteria and the immune system are mentioned, but it is just as important to shine a light on bacteria that suppress inflammation, like our faithful lactic acid bacteria, which have been shown to be beneficial to our brain and mental health. Lactic acid bacteria increase the concentration of anti-inflammatory cytokines in the blood and have even been shown to be able to repair a leaky blood-brain barrier caused by inflammatory substances.

Lactic acid bacteria are good for your brain and mental health.

# *A summary of chapter 2*

**The gut-brain axis**

- A silent dialogue occurs twenty-four seven between your gut and brain
- Most of this data traffic travels upward from the gut to the brain
- The brain is more reliant on information from our gut than the other way around.

**The gut—your second brain**

- The gut's nervous system consists of fifty to a hundred million nerve cells
- The gut's nervous system belongs to the autonomic nervous system
- The gut's nervous system is a high-performing security system
- The gut's nervous system consists of a sensory network of roughly 430 square feet.

**Bacteria—a critical part of the gut-brain axis**

- Trillions of bacteria take part in the dialogue between the gut and brain
- Bacteria communicate with their biochemical language (neurotransmitters and metabolites)
- Bacteria and the gut work together like a "pharmaceutical factory"
- Bacteria are vital to a normal development of the brain, especially during the first three years of life

**The gut, bacteria, and your emotions**

- Every emotion has an equivalent "facial expression" in the gut
- Bacteria in your gut can be affected by what you are thinking and feeling
- Stress can fuel harmful bacteria and reduce beneficial bacteria
- Stress can cause bacteria to transform stress hormones to more powerful versions of themselves.

**A lifelong symbiosis—humankind and bacteria**

- Our symbiotic contract with bacteria has existed for more than five hundred million years
- Bacteria prefer to live in mutual harmony with their human host
- Lifestyle factors (food, exercise, stress, etc.) affect this symbiotic contract

**"Bacteria-brain" map**

- Two chemical messengers: neurotransmitters and metabolites
- Two barriers: the gut barrier and blood-brain barrier
- Two main roads: the vagus nerve and blood circulation
- Two X-factors: food and stress (that affect gut-brain axis)
- Two healing substances: fiber (prebiotics) and good bacteria (probiotics)

**The gut—your own pharmaceutical factory**

- 90 percent of the body's serotonin is produced in the gut
- 50 percent of all dopamine is produced in the gut
- Bacteria produce short-chain fatty acids, such as butyric acid and acetate

CHAPTER 3

# The role of gut bacteria in our mental health and more

# *The dark epidemic of our time*

Next time you find yourself in a crowded place, maybe a train station, airport, or shopping mall, look around. One in six adults in the United States will experience depression at some point in their lives, and about one in fifteen will have experienced at least one major depressive episode in a given year. In Sweden, depression has become so common that nearly one in four Swedes are at some point in life affected by a depression so severe that it requires medical treatment. The truth is that over 350 million people around the world suffer from depression—a figure that is expected to rise. In addition, globally, depression is the main reason for a reduced work capacity. By 2020, the World Health Organization (WHO) believes that depression will surpass heart and cardiovascular diseases as the diagnosis that will be most costly to society. Similar to depression, anxiety is also spreading across the world like a plague. Across the world, around 275 million people are believed to suffer from anxiety disorders, an increase of 40 million in only ten years.

When it comes to stress, eight out of ten Americans say they frequently or sometimes encounter stress throughout the day. In Sweden, the number of people who suffer from serious stress has increased by over 100 percent in only ten years, a number that includes more and more children. Without a doubt, stress-related illnesses are an epidemic of our time, causing huge costs to society as well as suffering—both for the affected person and their loved ones. No one is immune.

What do we really mean by the term *mental health*? It is broad and vague, and there is really no established definition even though it is used in research and official contexts, as well as in our daily lives. The term encompasses everything, from a diagnosis of depression, anxiety disorder, and schizophrenia to just feeling mentally unwell (stress, grief, sleeping problems) without a diagnosis. While many people feel that a term like *psychological disorder* is too loaded and difficult to talk honestly about, most others find it easier to open up about *mental health* to discuss specific, well-defined mental health disorders as well as the issues that are more vague or broader in definition. Our struggle to get to the bottom of mental illness is all the more reason to unlock more clues to discover how we can reduce mental health suffering—and this is why new research on the role of gut bacteria in mental health is so exciting.

Apart from mental health, this chapter will also discuss the role gut bacteria plays in influencing the brain-related disorders Alzheimer's, Parkinson's, autism, and attention-deficit/hyperactivity disorder (ADHD).

I have chosen to discuss these common psychiatric and neurological disorders that affect many of us directly and indirectly at some stage in our lives. These diagnoses also reflect several age-groups over a life span—children (autism and ADHD), adults and teenagers (stress, depression, and anxiety), and the older generation (Alzheimer's and Parkinson's). I will start with stress-related illnesses (stress, depression, and anxiety), continue with degenerative illnesses that effect the elderly (Alzheimer's and Parkinson's), and finish off by looking at how far research on bacteria has come with regards to various neuropsychiatric disorders among children (autism and ADHD). One thing is for certain: our perspective on psychiatric and neurological disorders will be different when seen through the bacterial lens.

### The gut and mental health—nothing new

Even over a hundred years ago, a group of medical researchers saw that toxic conditions in the gut could cause mental health problems. Some doctors even suggested that signals from the gut to the brain could regulate emotional responses. Their studies and claims were soon dismissed. In the middle of the twentieth century, a "truth" was established that a psychological or emotional state can affect the gut, but not the other way around. For a long time, it was thought that the connection between the brain and gut was one-way—the connection was mainly studied from the point of view of digestion, where mental stress could affect digestive functions such as in IBS, but an imbalance in gut flora could not in turn cause mental health problems.

Research has thankfully moved on and there are many things that point to the fact that the link between the gut and the brain goes both ways.

### Gut bacteria and mental health—big news

This two-way communication between the gut and brain concerns a lot more than just the overseeing of our digestive functions. It wasn't that long ago that researchers first discovered that gut bacteria directly influence stress-related behavior and play an important role in developing anxiety and depression. The gut and gut bacteria have been shown to have an effect on mood, motivation, behavior, and cognitive functioning. behavior

This two-way communication is a complex and multifaceted process involving many of the body's systems, including the nervous system, immune system, and hormonal system. Everything is connected.

## *The role of gut bacteria in stress, anxiety, and depression*

The activities that occur in our brain when we suffer from stress, anxiety, or depression have been shown to be fairly similar to one another. This is why stress, anxiety, and depression are often lumped together as stress-related disorders, or *SAD* as I call them (not to be confused with seasonal affective disorder syndrome or the standard American diet). SAD is the most common form of mental health problems among teenagers and adults.

In small doses, stress now and then is harmless, but too much for too long can cause a chronic state of stress that in turn can lead to anxiety disorders such as panic disorder and different phobias. Continued anxiety can also lead to depression.

We know that groundbreaking research has shown that gut bacteria play a deciding factor in SAD, so let's take a closer look at this, starting with stress.

## Stress and gut bacteria

Stress affects more and more people today. In America, stress is cited as a major contributing factor to the six leading causes of death: cancer, coronary heart disease, accidental injuries, respiratory disorders, cirrhosis of the liver, and suicide. In Sweden, around a third of all illnesses in women between the ages 35 and 49 are stress-related. Stress also affects younger people—since 2006, there has been a 142 percent increase in the number of children aged five to nine who have been diagnosed with stress reactions.

Stress has positive effects up to a certain breaking point, and anything after that causes damage. The positioning of this breaking point is related to several factors (genetic vulnerability, environment, illness, events, etc.). Research now shows that the composition of your gut flora can affect your stress threshold and how you respond to stress. The opposite is also the case—stress affects the composition of your gut flora.

So, what is stress? Essentially, stress is a requirement for survival. Everyone experiences stress at times—the stress of deadlines, the stress of having children, holiday stress, daily stress, and so on. Stress has become such an integral part of our lives that most people just see it a natural occurrence.

Of all the definitions of stress that exist, the following has caught my eye: a state of disharmony or a threat to homeostasis. By homeostasis, I mean the stable equilibrium that all biological systems aim to maintain within its surroundings. Take body temperature, for example: your body constantly regulates several organs against the surrounding environment to keep the temperature at 37 degrees. Too low or too high a temperature can lead to death. Stress occurs when the body's equilibrium is threatened. Stress is, in other words, evolution's response to threats against our homeostasis.

#### ACUTE STRESS IS OKAY

Even though stress is usually understood in a negative context, we are made to occasionally handle acute stress during shorter periods of time as long as this is layered with periods of recuperation and rest. When the body is exposed to long-term stress without rest, it then becomes harmful. If you are stressed for too long, high amounts of the stress hormone, cortisol, can shrink the hippocampus in your brain, which, bearing in mind that our hippocampus is important to memory and orientation, is not a good thing. Sadly, our ancient stress system (also called the *HPA-axis*) can't distinguish between real-life threats (a lion attack) and false alarms (no one likes your latest Instagram photo), and your stress system releases stress hormones as soon as you experience an event, a person, or a situation that is seen to be negative.

#### CHRONIC STRESS IS NOT OKAY!

If this goes on for too long and happens too often, stress can open up the road to chronic imbalance and cause more illness. Symptoms of ongoing stress can be physical (headache, stomach problems, sleep problems), emotional (mood swings, feelings of loneliness), pertaining to thoughts (negative self-image) or behavioral (eating, substance abuse). It is also common to have several stress symptoms at the same time. Stress symptoms and what causes stress varies from person to person and even from moment to moment. Long-term or chronic stress can easily turn to anxiety and depression, which affect the gut flora negatively in a vicious circle.

#### STRESS FEEDS HARMFUL GUT BACTERIA

Stress hormones like noradrenaline can drastically change your gut flora by increasing the number of harmful gut bacteria and reducing the amount of beneficial lactic acid bacteria. This is how it works: stress causes the adrenal glands to release the stress hormone noradrenaline (which, among other things, makes the heart beat faster and increases blood pressure). In turn, noradrenaline stimulates the growth of harmful bacteria. In addition, noradrenaline has been shown to make these bacteria more aggressive, increasing their chance of survival. Some bacteria can even transform the noradrenaline that's already floating around to a more harmful type (adrenaline), which intensifies the harmful effects of stress. As if this wasn't enough, the harmful effects stress has on gut flora can even change several critical signaling paths between the gut and brain, contributing to the development of depression and anxiety disorders.

In summary: short-term stress can be positive, even in our gut, when acute stress increases the production of stomach acid, which increases the chance of harmful bacteria dying before they reach our intestines. However, the benefits turn to disadvantages as soon as acute stress becomes chronic. Stress hormones remain at an unhealthily high level in the blood and can harm the body in different ways. Stress in small doses is not harmful, but overdosing on stress over a longer period of time can get really dangerous—especially for your gut flora and brain.

#### STRESS LOOSENS YOUR GUT (LEAKY GUT SYNDROME)

Stress hormones reduce the width of the gut's mucous membrane, causing leakage. This in turn makes it possible for toxic bacteria to pass through and get better access to the gut's immune system, which is immediately activated, resulting in increased inflammation. This chain (stress–leaky gut–bacteria–inflammation) has been shown to be connected to depression and many other brain-related illnesses. Simply put, stress has a harmful effect on your gut-brain axis.

#### STRESS EARLY ON IN LIFE SHAPES YOUR GUT FLORA

The harmful effects of stress on gut flora seem to transfer from mother to child. One study showed how women who experienced high levels of stress during pregnancy had children who had a gut flora with less beneficial bacteria than those who were not exposed to high stress. These children also had other health issues, such as allergies and food and gut problems. One (cruel) way to research the effect of stress on gut flora is to separate the child from its mother early in life. A study from 2015 showed that mice that were removed from their mothers as newborns still had a high level of the stress hormone cortisol as an adult. Several similar studies show that early separation from the mother creates long-lasting changes in gut flora, stress profiles, and behavior.

#### BACTERIA REGULATE STRESS SYMPTOMS

The exciting thing in these studies is that regular lactic acid bacteria that can be found in yogurt and kimchi was shown to reduce stress hormones in the mice. In fact, all abnormalities in the brain completely disappeared when the traumatized mice that had been separated from their mother were exposed to lactic acid bacteria early in life. Researchers now believe that colonizing bacteria immediately after birth kick-starts the important mechanisms in the brain that handle stress and emotional behavior. Apart from the mice who had been separated early from their mothers, mice who didn't have any bacteria were shown to be very sensitive to stress; they also displayed "asocial" behaviors. But when lactic acid was introduced, even these stress symptoms disappeared.

This groundbreaking study from 2004 showed that it was enough to give mice that were free from bacteria the lactic acid *B. infantis* to calm the brain. Researchers were also fascinated to find out that this goes both ways. When researchers transplanted poo from calm mice to the hyper-stressed bacteria-free mice, the stressed mice calmed down, but worryingly enough it also worked when poo from the hyper-stressed mice were transferred to the calm ones, causing the previously calm mice to display stress and anxiety-related behaviors.

## Anxiety, depression, and gut bacteria

Anxiety and depression are closely related and might be considered cousins. As you know, long-term anxiety can turn into depression, and many people suffer from anxiety and depression at the same time. Anxiety is therefore one of the symptoms in a depression diagnosis. That's why it is common for antidepressants to be prescribed together with medicines that combat anxiety. People with anxiety and depression also share several physiological conditions, such as stomach problems; sleep problems; increased inflammation; lower levels of the brain's growth hormone (BDNF), especially in the area relating to memory; high levels of cortisol; a heightened stress response; and an increased leaky gut. You could say that the main difference between anxiety and depression is that anxiety is about an excessive worry and fear of the future, while depression is more of a feeling of meaninglessness and hopelessness. If a person affected by anxiety is worried about "the end of the world," a depressed person feels that "the world has already ended."

In this section, we'll take a closer look at new research that explores the important relationships among anxiety, depression, and our gut bacteria; we'll also see how you can improve your mental health.

### ANXIETY—A NATURAL STRESS REACTION

Similar to stress, anxiety is a natural reaction, and experiencing anxiety doesn't necessarily mean that anything is "wrong" with you. The stress symptoms you experience when you have anxiety are caused by your body's reactions to something that appears threatening. The body gets ready to handle the situation by increasing the amount of adrenaline and other stress hormones in the blood. Symptoms of anxiety show themselves through an increase in stress—muscles contract, the heart beats faster, and breathing becomes more intensive. It is also common to have problems breathing, the feeling of being choked, difficulty in swallowing, stomach problems, chest pains, dizziness, and nausea. On the psychological side, anxiety can appear as problems in concentration;

exhaustion; feeling detached; or fears of going crazy, losing control, or dying. Often an anxiety attack will pass by itself, but when anxiety remains and causes so much suffering that it drastically reduces a person's quality of life, it then becomes a psychiatric illness, falling under the broader category of anxiety disorders.

### DEPRESSION—MORE DEADLY THAN TRAFFIC

What are the signs of depression? The typical symptoms are a low mood, feeling empty, feeling that life is meaningless, and having problems finding joy in everyday life. It's normal for us to feel low sometimes, and the feeling usually passes by itself; but when low mood continues over several weeks or months and causes a great reduction in a person's quality of life, it becomes depression. In other words, it's a bit tricky to know exactly where the boundary lies between a natural feeling of being low and a psychiatric disorder. In addition, there is a broad spectrum of depressions with a myriad of different symptoms, such as low mood, feeling guilty, sadness, anxiety, sleeplessness, tiredness, lack of energy, meaninglessness, suicidal thoughts, aching body, constipation, menstrual disturbances, reduced sexual appetite, sleep and concentration problems, reduced memory, lack of appetite, and so on. Usually, depressed people struggle to handle their jobs, school life, and everyday tasks. If it goes too far, depression can lead to thoughts of suicide, as well as the act of suicide. The fact is that depression is the singular largest risk factor of suicide. Did you know that, on average, 129 people take their own lives per day in the United States? In Sweden, five people die from suicide every day, which is five times more than the number of people who die in traffic.

### IS DEPRESSION A CHEMICAL IMBALANCE OF THE BRAIN . . .

It is believed that changes in the balance between different neurotransmitters in the brain cause depression. Depression is most typically linked to reduced levels of serotonin.



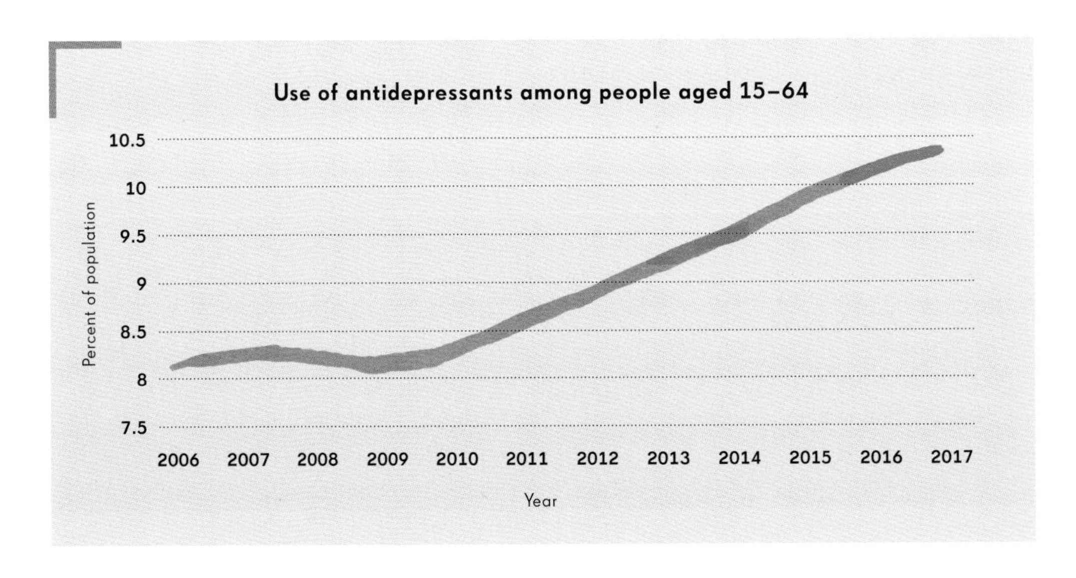

Antidepressants therefore work to increase the levels of serotonin in the brain. The problem with medicines that raise serotonin levels (SSRIs), such as Prozac, is that they can take several weeks before any positive effects start to show. Until then, symptoms may even get worse and side effects may result. The fact is, if the issue was only about raising serotonin levels in the brain, these medications should have an immediate effect.

Instead, many researchers now believe that serotonin stimulates the creation of new brain cells (neurogenesis) and new connections (synaptic plasticity), and it is this that repairs a "damaged" brain. However, neurogenesis has been shown to be less effective in depressed people than in others. To repair and build new brain cells is a gradual change that can take a few weeks, which would explain the delayed effect of the antidepressants. Fortunately, new groundbreaking research shows that gut bacteria seem to be involved in the creation of new brain cells, again shining a light on the central role bacteria plays in our brain.

### ... OR INFLAMMATION IN THE BRAIN?

The notion that depression might be caused by an imbalance in the brain is being challenged by a radically different viewpoint as new research is showing that depression can be linked to inflammation in the brain. The findings can be summarized like this: inflammation in the body can propagate inflammation to the head, and the more inflammatory substances that are whizzing around the body, the deeper the depression seems to get.

Some studies have been extra remarkable—one such study showed that brain tissue was inflamed in deeply depressed patients who had lacked treatment for a long period. Researchers discovered that the level of inflammation was 33 percent higher in some regions of the brain compared to patients who had been medicated. Many researchers therefore suggest that some cases of depression can be the result of inflammation. One interesting discovery was that nervous cell inflammation could be halted using antidepressants. As a result, researchers are currently looking at the possibility of using inflammation-inhibiting medication to treat patients with depression. Hardly surprising then is that depression is sometimes known as *neuroinflammation*, that is to say, inflammation of the brain.

### DEPRESSION AND INFLAMMATION-INDUCING GUT FLORA

What do the relationships among depression, inflammation, and our gut bacteria look like? When researchers gave healthy mice an injection with inflammation-causing LPS, they immediately developed depression-like syndromes. The rogue in this drama is LPS, bad bacteria's firebomb we learned about earlier (see p. 26). What do these firebombs do again? Well, when bad firebomb bacteria die in large numbers, they release a large amount of LPS and other substances that contribute to a leaky gut. In addition, LPS production is increased by inflammation-causing substances in the gut. The fact that people with depression often exhibit inflamed and porous gut walls is thought to be due to the large amounts of LPS in their blood. Once released into the bloodstream, LPS particles can move through the critical blood-brain barrier in your brain, and when they reach the inside of your holy organ, they inflame the brain.

Apart from depression, researchers believe that inflammation can also lead to Alzheimer's later on in life. When compared to healthy people, LPS levels have been shown to be a lot higher in people with depression and three times as high in people with Alzheimer's. Some researchers even suggest that people who have suffered depression run double the risk of suffering from Alzheimer's or substantial cognitive impairments. Science is currently looking into whether even low-level inflammation can directly cause cognitive impairments.

#### DOES DEPRESSION HAVE A BACTERIAL SIGNATURE?

The question everyone is asking today is whether depression has a bacterial signature. But even if scientists haven't yet found a unique bacterial signature for depression, it has been shown in several studies that the gut flora in people with depression contain more of the bacterial genus Alistipes. Alistipes has also been linked to IBS and exhaustion. What then does the connection between the Alistipes bacteria and depression look like?

For the body to be able to produce the happy molecule serotonin, it needs access to the amino acid tryptophan. But with Alistipes present, tryptophan is converted into the bad-smelling substance indole instead (the same substance that gives feces its unpleasant odor). People with depression have been shown to have higher levels of indole and lower levels of serotonin; however, the research is not yet complete. While the chase to discover the unique bacterial signature for depression is ongoing, more scientists believe that it is less important to focus on an exact bacterial signature and more important to highlight diversity and have large enough amounts of beneficial bacteria, such as lactic acid bacteria.

### How you can protect your brain

If you were raised on a typical Western diet, it is likely that you are walking around with a high level of inflammation-inducing firebomb bacteria like Firmicutes in your gut. The good news is that you can reduce the number of firebomb bacteria by consuming foods that contain probiotics and prebiotics.

#### PROBIOTICS: CAN LACTIC ACID BACTERIA REDUCE MENTAL HEALTH PROBLEMS?

Do you eat probiotics? It is a trendy supplement these days, and rightly so! Probiotics are defined by the WHO as "living microorganisms that in large enough doses have a positive health effect on its host." Probiotics usually consist of regular lactic acid bacteria from the *Bifidobacterium* and *Lactobacillus* groups, which have a healing effect on both the gut and brain. You can find plenty of lactic acid bacteria in fermented food like yogurt, kimchi, and kombucha. A good health tip is to start eating more fermented foods—and you can find out how to make your very own kimchi and kombucha in chapter 5.

Many animal studies have shown that probiotic lactic acid bacteria radically reduce symptoms of stress and depression. For example, stress symptoms are greatly reduced when severely stressed mice were given *B. infantis*. In fact, the lactic acid bacteria create gamma-Aminobutyric acid (GABA), which calms the nervous system.

Even studies on humans have shown that lactic acid bacteria reduce stress and anxiety, and researchers could even see these clear changes in the brain with the help of fMRI. These initial studies were conducted on healthy volunteers, and scientists believe that the effect would be even greater in people diagnosed with mental health disorders. While awaiting more large-scale studies on humans, discussions are growing around the medicinal capacity of probiotics to treat mental health disorders, and an increasing number of scientists believe that health care will soon introduce "probiotics on prescription." The question that also arises is how much lactic acid bacteria would be needed to reach a possible medicinal effect.

#### PREBIOTICS: IS FIBER AS EFFECTIVE AS MEDICATION?

If probiotics are the good bacteria, then prebiotics are the food and nutrition for the good bacteria. *Prebiotics* is a group term for indigestible, complex carbohydrates (fiber) that act as nourishment for our good bacteria, probiotics, to stimulate their growth. An important group is oligosaccharides, which are found in breast milk, fruit, and vegetables (see pp. 92–93).

Studies have actually shown that oligosaccharides can reduce stress, anxiety, and depression. In one study, the saliva from healthy people was measured in the morning when the level of the stress hormone cortisol is considered to be the highest. After having eating oligosaccharides for a few weeks, scientists found lower levels of cortisol. In addition, the participants showed reduced vigilance toward negative stimuli, which is reflective of anxiety-reducing and antidepressant effects.

In a more drastic experiment, mice were fed galactooligosaccharides (GOS) via breast milk from humans prior to being exposed to stress. It was shown that the GOS protected the mice from damage to the central nervous system through stress, whereas mice that had not received breast milk showed anxiety-related behaviors and fewer brain cells in the hippocampus. Last but not least, a notable study from Oxford showed that healthy volunteers who took oligosaccharides reduced their levels of anxiety in a way that was equivalent to taking antidepressants and anxiety-reducing Valium! Summarily, preliminary research indicates that prebiotic fiber could have a stress- and anxiety-reducing effect. So, if you are feeling a bit low, try to get some GOS inside you. More information about GOS and prebiotics can be found on pp. 92–93. Of course, it also goes without saying that despite this fantastic news, you should not just stop any medication you're talking without consulting your doctor.

#### ANTIBIOTICS: DEPRESSION IS MADE WORSE BY PENICILLIN

In animal studies, antibiotics have been shown to lead to increased depression and reduced cognitive functioning. Antibiotics even reduced newly produced brain cells in areas of the brain that are important for, among other things, learning, memory, and emotional regulation. The amounts of feel-good molecules like oxytocin, vasopressin, and a turnover of tryptophan (the raw material of serotonin) was also reduced. Interestingly enough, these negative effects could be reduced by probiotics or exercise. However, the results are mixed with antibiotics—scientists have also seen no signs of anxiety-type symptoms after treatment with antibiotics, probably because the antibiotics got rid of bad bacteria. But in general, it is believed that antibiotics are harmful to gut flora and that they worsen depression.

#### FOOD: WESTERN FOOD INFLAMES THE BRAIN

Apart from antibiotics, there are also dangerous foods that can worsen your mental health. The bad guys are mainly Western foods, which have a high percentage of animal fat and lots of sugar that drastically increase stress hormones and inflammation-producing bacteria. Even though the link between fatty foods and stress has been common knowledge for a while, it has only been recently that we've discovered that gut flora is a deciding factor in this mechanism (see chapter 4).

Stress also gives you an involuntary craving for food that is high in calories. This means that a mixed cocktail of saturated fats and foods high in sugars plus stress is a toxic combination that fuels inflammation-enhancing bacteria in a vicious cycle. Recently, researchers have found inflammatory markers inside the brain's hippocampus as a direct result of stress and a bad diet. Stress and food are two factors that affect how your gut flora, and subsequently your gut-brain axis, feel. If you want to prevent stress, anxiety, and depression, eat an anti-inflammatory diet that is as gut-friendly as possible. You can read all about how to strengthen your brain and gut flora with food in chapters 4 and 5.



## *The role of gut bacteria in Alzheimer's and Parkinson's*

Let's leave stress-related illnesses and move on to age-related illnesses.

We know that gut flora have been shown to play a huge part in Alzheimer's disease and Parkinson's disease, which are neurodegenerative illnesses that occur when the nervous system slowly atrophies. Primarily, it is the nerve cells in the brain that break down and die, causing important functions to be reduced or even stop, and in time leading to devastating damage.

Alzheimer's and Parkinson's are sneaky degenerative processes because they normally begin long before any symptoms appear. New research shows that gut bacteria can play an important role in neurodegenerative Illnesses, and we will take a closer look, starting with the most common form of dementia, Alzheimer's.

### Alzheimer's disease and gut bacteria

Did you know that every four seconds, someone in the world is diagnosed with dementia? Try counting this aloud to yourself (one, two, three, four . . . BAM), and you'll see what a ticking time bomb it is. In fact, as many as half of all people over the age of eighty-five are at risk of suffering from dementia, and even now every fifth Swede over the age of eighty has dementia. In the United States, five million people are currently living with dementia, and a large demographic leap will come after 2020, when baby boomers

**Soki Choi reflects on the gut's own pharmaceutical factory**

Psychiatric health problems are a cash cow. In the West, consumption of antidepressants has doubled since 2000. In Sweden, over 10 percent of the population takes antidepressants and this number is on the rise, especially among young people where the use of these medications has almost doubled. Whenever I read the marketing reports of pharmaceutical companies, I'm struck by their cynical tone, where mental health problems among young people are portrayed as a great "marketing opportunity."

That's why I welcome all the research that has shown that cheap and simple methods like as exercise, meditation, and food can have the same effect as antidepressants. Sometimes it can be enough just to run for 45 minutes three times a week to get the medicinal effect as a drug after a few weeks. Hopefully, we can soon bring the knowledge of the health benefits of fiber and bacteria straight onto the medical stage when it comes to treating patients.

Imagine if you're able to start preventative measures early enough with exercise and healthy food, and lower your risk of becoming a victim of mental health disorders, where you'll be forced to take medicine with scary side effects after the fact. Wouldn't that be great?

born in the 1940s will reach their eighties. It is estimated that one out of every six women and one out of every ten men will develop dementia if they live past the age of fifty-five. In 2015, the worldwide economic cost of dementia is believed to be approximately $818 billion.

Alzheimer's is the most common form of dementia. Typically, the first symptoms appear after sixty years of age, before developing into the disease after age eighty-five. Age is without a doubt the largest "risk factor" in someone getting Alzheimer's.

#### PLAQUE IN THE BRAIN

Alzheimer's is an inconsiderate disease where you gradually lose your brain cells, leading to the loss of bodily function and a sped-up death. Two proteins—tau and beta-amyloid—clump together and form plaque in the brain, although we don't know why this happens. How does Alzheimer's present in a person? Typically, it starts with loss of memory, such as forgetfulness and struggling to find words.

Other symptoms include aimlessly wandering around and getting lost, as well as picking up things and putting them back in places where you forget them. Compulsive repetitive behaviors such as opening and closing doors continually are a further irritation for people in the surrounding environment. When anxious cries, shouts, and aggression are added to the list, it starts to get extra difficult for caretakers. As the illness continues, the body will start to malfunction, and there may be difficulty in controlling urination and even defecation in more severe cases. In addition, symptoms such as stiffness, cramps, and involuntary muscle spasms can plague the sufferer toward the end. The effects of Alzheimer's are great and go beyond the individual.



#### INFLAMMATION-PROMOTING GUT FLORA

For several decades, researchers believed that Alzheimer's was caused by clumps of protein building up in the brain and that inflammation was just a symptom of Alzheimer's. But new research shows that inflammation is more of a cause of Alzheimer's, which has turned the scientific world upside down. Researchers now believe that symptoms of Alzheimer's can be reduced by eating anti-inflammatory food or taking anti-inflammatory medication—and this is where gut flora comes in.

The first study on humans that examined the link among Alzheimer's, inflammation, and gut flora appeared in 2016. It was an Italian study that divided a 150 people into three groups. One group consisted of people with Alzheimer's, the other group suffered memory problems (but without the typical plaque in the brain that indicates Alzheimer's), and the last group was a healthy control group. The people with Alzheimer's did not have any genetic predisposition for Alzheimer's (genetic predisposition is a large risk factor). By comparing the feces and blood samples from the groups, researchers were able to confirm that those with Alzheimer's had a different setup of gut bacteria when compared with the other two control groups—they had an overflow of the inflammation-causing bacteria escherichia/shigella, a bacteria that had been shown in previous studies to cause the body to produce cytokines. The blood samples of those with Alzheimer's also contained a lot more of these inflammation-causing cytokines. Researchers could also confirm that they had a much lower rate of the good anti-inflammatory bacteria *Eubacterium rectale*, which is known to produce the beneficial inflammation-reducing butyric acid. Researchers also saw a lower quantity of inflammation-reducing substances than normal. Even if the sample of bacteria was somewhat limited, this research is considered groundbreaking. For the first time, a clinical study pointed to the fact the composition of gut flora could be an important factor that drives Alzheimer's.

During 2017, the highly respected journal *Nature* published several articles on Alzheimer's and gut flora. One of the studies showed that the diversity of bacteria in the gut flora was greatly reduced in people with Alzheimer's when compared to a healthy control group. Without getting fixated on specific bacteria, the main message was that Alzheimer's seem to go hand in hand with an inflammatory-enhancing gut flora of reduced variety.

#### PROBIOTICS: LACTIC ACID BACTERIA REDUCES THE PLAQUE TYPICAL OF ALZHEIMER'S

The amazing news is that it has been shown that lactic acid bacteria can reduce the symptoms of Alzheimer's. In 2014, a study showed that a cocktail of eight probiotic bacteria could regulate genes that control age-related changes in old mice. They had less brain inflammation and a better memory and plasticity thanks to their bacterial cocktail. Another study from 2017 tested a different probiotic cocktail on mice with symptoms similar to those of Alzheimer's in its early stages, and showed that the neural pathway and brain damage eventually repaired and the plaque typical of Alzheimer's had reduced because of the lactic acid bacteria. Cognitive impairment in these mice also reduced when compared to the control group. These studies point to the fact that the exact composition of lactic acid bacteria is not the deciding factor and that the ingredients can vary. The important thing seems to be to introduce living probiotic bacteria in large enough doses inside you.

At the end of 2016, a notable study on sixty people with severe Alzheimer's was presented. The subjects were divided into two groups, where one drank a milk cocktail with probiotic lactic acid bacteria from the *Lactobacillus* and *Bifidobacterium* groups and the other group drank regular milk. After twelve weeks the researchers compared the subjects' cognitive abilities. They found that patients with Alzheimer's who had drunk the milk with probiotics had increased their cognitive ability by up to 30 percent. Even if this was a randomized, double blind, and placebo-controlled study, it obviously needs to be repeated several more times and in larger settings. That being said, if "normal" lactic acid bacteria have been shown to drastically improve the brain in people with severe Alzheimer's, it would be, to put it mildly, groundbreaking.

#### PREBIOTICS: FIBER ENHANCES A DRASTICALLY IMPAIRED MEMORY

Prebiotic fiber acts like food to butyric acid–producing bacteria. A mountain of studies have shown that butyric acid has anti-inflammatory properties that inhibit the growth of cancer cells in the large intestine. In 2011, two groups of scientists took this to the next level in the context of Alzheimer's and showed that butyric acid can even improve age-related memory functions that are becoming greatly impaired. The experiments were conducted on lab mice, which is often the case in research in its early stages. For your gut bacteria to produce butyric acid, you need to feed them prebiotic fiber (such as that found in fruit, vegetables, etc.). Above all, they like the prebiotic resistant starch, which can be found in potato flour and even cold pasta, rice, and potato. Prebiotic fiber is also plentiful in kimchi.

#### ANTIBIOTICS REDUCE THE PLAQUE TYPICAL OF ALZHEIMER'S

Surprisingly enough, antibiotics have been shown to have positive effects in the context of Alzheimer's. In a study from 2016, researchers discovered that after ingesting antibiotics, the amount of typical plaque in the brain of mice that had been given symptoms similar to those of Alzheimer's were reduced. In addition, their immune response was improved, and the progression of the disease was halted after the gut flora had changed. Researchers were unable to answer definitively if it was the effect of the antibiotics that had knocked out harmful bacteria or if it was the new gut flora that had benefited the mice. The link between a change in gut flora and reductions of the plaque typical of Alzheimer's was established, nonetheless. Even if our modern-day overuse of antibiotics is not healthy, this study points to the fact that for people with an unhealthy gut flora—as in the case of someone with Alzheimer's—controlled antibiotics can promote a healthier gut flora and even halt the progress of the disease. In light of the one-sided criticism antibiotics often get, this is a good example that shows that something is never just good or bad but always dependent on the context. If the doctors of tomorrow were to treat a serious neurodegenerative illness such as Alzheimer's with the same medicine you might get for a sinus or throat infection, it would be groundbreaking. Not too long ago, this concept would have been laughable, provocative, and unthinkable—but not today.

**ALZHEIMER'S AND THE HYGIENE HYPOTHESIS**

In the Western world, our cleanliness culture has taken a lot of criticism for being the bane of all modern illnesses, such as allergies and asthma. Can we also add Alzheimer's to the list? Researchers have for a long time wondered why the rate of Alzheimer's varies so much around the world. A group of scientists from Cambridge collected data from 192 countries and lay them neatly along two axes. There was a clear linear correlation—less developed countries with lower hygiene standards had a lower occurrence of Alzheimer's while more developed countries with higher hygiene standards had higher occurrences of Alzheimer's. Even though it was just a correlation and many other factors could be considered, the researchers allowed themselves to draw the brave conclusion that the hygiene standards in the Western world, which tend to be more developed, increase the risk of Alzheimer's. However, before you drag your poor grandma or grandpa out into the woods, let's consider the theory of Martin Blaser from New York University. Dr. Blaser has studied gut flora for over thirty years, and he believes that the overuse of antibiotics in combination along with the consumption of processed food is the biggest culprit that causes Alzheimer's. Plus, there are plenty of bacteria in dirt and soil in our surroundings that do not add anything of value to humans. Dr. Blaser is therefore skeptical of the parents who feed their children soil to strengthen their immune system, or, as he says, "The microbes in dirt have evolved for soil, not for us."

**PARKINSON'S DISEASE AND GUT BACTERIA**

After Alzheimer's, Parkinson's disease is the most common neurodegenerative disease. Around the world, around 6 million people suffer from Parkinson's at the moment. In the United States, nearly one million people will be living with Parkinson's by 2020, and approximately sixty thousand are diagnosed with the disease each year. In Sweden, around twenty thousand people have Parkinson's, and every year, two thousand more get a diagnosis. People over fifty years old are mainly affected, and in those over age sixty, the disease appears in 100 of 10,000 people. Dementia and depression also often appear together with Parkinson's.

**Soki Choi reflects on the relevance of studies that use animals**

The link between gut flora and the brain is a new field of research, and as with all research in its early stages, experiments are often done on animals for ethical reasons. The question then arises: to what extent can we apply the results from mice to humans? The truth is that mice can't really get Alzheimer's, so what researchers do is artificially create symptoms similar to those of Alzheimer's in mice. It may not be ideal, but it is effective when they can't experiment on humans for ethical reasons. In the defense of researchers, the basic mechanisms in cells are so stable and conserved by millions of years of evolution that there is minimal difference between the species. And the more elementary the process, the further we can move away from humans to experiment on another species and still yield applicable results. This is why researchers can understand human cell division by studying yeast, or understand the brain of embryos by studying fruit flies (however banal that might sound). Leading gut scientists believe we can absolutely draw parallels from animals since the cells that surround our guts are very similar in all mammals. Hopefully, this will make it easier for us to embrace the results of these earlier studies.

Since we are living longer, the number of people afflicted will increase in the future. Despite decades of intensive research, we still don't know why a person develops Parkinson's. We do however know that anyone can get it and that age is a big risk factor. It is also more common for men to get Parkinson's than it is for women. There is no known cure or medication that can halt the process. Like Alzheimer's, Parkinson's is one of medicine's great mysteries.

#### A TREACHEROUS PROCESS

Parkinson's is probably best known for its three main motor symptoms: uncontrollable tremors, stiff muscles, and slow movement. With Parkinson's, the person loses essential brain cells that produce dopamine. You probably know that dopamine is the brain's reward substance, but did you know that it also controls our voluntary and fine motor movements? That is why people with Parkinson's struggle to get moving. There are no tests that can see if you have Parkinson's, but the doctor will likely diagnose a patient from the symptoms shown. The disease is treacherous as it starts slowly, long before any of the visible tremors appear. The first symptoms might be constipation, loss of a sense of smell and sight, sleeplessness (usually with vivid nightmares), concentration difficulties, and depression. These early symptoms often occur years before the classic symptoms of Parkinson's appear. In contrast to the obvious motor symptoms of Parkinson's, these other symptoms are often not diagnosed or treated. The suspicion that one might suffer from Parkinson's is usually first triggered when an arm, leg, or both start to shake for a bit each day, while the person becomes slightly clumsy and starts to find writing or snapping their fingers difficult. However, by then the disease has already gone so far that irreversible brain damage has already occurred. This dangerous process is very slow and It usually takes decades. In the end, all conscious movement is affected, even speech and the ability to swallow.

#### PLAQUE IN THE BRAIN AGAIN

Similar to what happens in Alzheimer's, plaque-like structures build in the brain of someone with Parkinson's. This plaque is called *Lewy bodies*. They are made of alpha-synuclein, and they cause essential dopamine-producing cells to die. Why the plaque builds in the brain is unknown, and so far research has pointed to the somewhat hollow explanation of: "it can be due to a combination of genes, aging, and various environmental and lifestyle factors." What we do know is that where a similar loss of cells happens naturally with aging, in Parkinson's, cells degenerate a lot quicker. There is no cure to stop the disease's progression, only medications that increase the levels of dopamine and eases the symptoms. Sadly, the medications stop being effective after a short period of time, but don't fret—recent discoveries have been made in research into Parkinson's, and guess which direction they are going? You're right: the gut and gut flora.

#### PLAQUE IN THE GUT

Constipation and bloating are typical early symptoms of Parkinson's, which can occur ten years before the typical tremors begin. Approximately 80 percent of all people with Parkinson's also have constipation, which is why researchers and doctors have started to notice early symptoms in the gut.

In an American study from 2016, researchers discovered the typical plaque associated with Parkinson's in the gut of patients with Parkinson's. Compared with healthy people, these patients also have a lot more leakage in the gut and higher levels of harmful bacterial residual products, which also means they have more harmful bacteria. As you know, bacterial toxins start a cascade of inflammation in the body, which can reach the brain. Many believe that a combination of oxidative stress, bacterial toxins, and a leaky gut can promote the buildup of plaque in both the gut and brain in people with Parkinson's. With the discovery of typical plaque associated with Parkinson's in the gut, researchers suspect that the gut might even be where Parkinson's begins. If this is the case, it would clarify the strange coincidence of stomach and gut problems that can be seen in so many patients with Parkinson's.

#### THE FLORA OF PEOPLE WITH PARKINSON'S TEEMS WITH BAD BACTERIA

A growing number of scientific studies show a clear link between Parkinson's and dysbiosis, which is an imbalance in the gut flora with an excess of bad bacterial species. Independent studies have been conducted in several parts of the world that also show that patients with Parkinson's have a clearly different gut flora than healthy people. In what way the gut flora differs in healthy people seems to be dependent on the region, which is why it has not been possible to ascertain which bacteria are typical in the gut flora of someone with Parkinson's. There is probably not just one set of "Parkinson's" flora but several variants depending on where in the world you live and what you eat. The bottom line is that the gut flora is marked by an excess of bad bacteria and a deficiency in good bacteria. What wasn't clear to the researchers was if the "sick" gut flora is the *cause* of Parkinson's or the *consequence* of the disease. This confusion might be clarified by the study presented in the next section.

#### GUT BACTERIA KICK-START PARKINSON'S

In a celebrated study, a group of mice were injected with gut bacteria from people with Parkinson's, which led to the mice showing classic "Parkinson's" symptoms. "This convinced us that it is gut bacteria that regulates and even starts Parkinson's symptoms," said Timothy Sampson, one of the scientists. Researchers suggest that certain gut bacteria release poisonous chemicals that reach and initiate brain damage via the gut's nervous system. This aligns well with studies that have shown that farmers who come into contact with poisonous pesticides are more likely to get Parkinson's than others. Whether the poison comes from within or outside, gut bacteria seems to play a decisive role in the development of the disease.

You can't always apply the results of studies that were conducted on animals to humans. If larger studies on humans also show that Parkinson's can be kick-started by gut bacteria, it would be a medical breakthrough. Firstly, the composition of a person's gut flora would provide a clear sign of Parkinson's. Secondly, Parkinson's could be discovered long before the familiar tremors appear and the brain damage has already begun. Future treatment methods can manipulate the gut flora early on in high-risk people (such as the elderly). Lastly, neurodegenerative brain disease could be treated like gastrointestinal diseases, which, if anything, would be revolutionary. That gut bacteria have been shown to play a central role in Parkinson's has not only surprised the world of science but also provided the older generation with hope and the message that if you have a healthy gut, you might be able to prevent Parkinson's. While waiting for bigger studies to be conducted, you have nothing to lose by looking after your gut flora right now, especially in light of the fact that Parkinson's and Alzheimer's develop over time.

## *The role of gut bacteria in autism and ADHD*

Finally, we turn to the role of gut bacteria in two psychiatric diagnoses normally given during childhood—autism and ADHD. Both autism and ADHD belong to the group called *neuropsychiatric disorders*—the brain and nervous system process information and impressions in a different way compared to most people. It doesn't necessary mean anything negative, but it often causes problems in social contexts. What is exciting is the news that gut bacteria appear to play a large role even when it comes to the development of neuropsychiatric disorders.

We will take a closer look at these links and begin with the neuropsychiatric disorder that researchers have gotten the furthest with: autism.

#### AUTISM AND GUT BACTERIA

Autistic spectrum disorder (ASD) is a broad term for diagnoses comprising the whole spectrum, from severe autism to high-functioning Asperger's syndrome. These diagnoses have in common that the person displays limitation in three areas, the so-called *triad of impairments*: (1) social interaction, (2) social communication, and (3) specific atypical behavior/perception. Even self-harming is common where autistic people might hit themselves in the face or bite their hands when they are stressed or happy. People with a milder form of autism, for example Asperger's, can have relatively normal conversations and therefore be considered normal or even high-functioning, but they still struggle to understand and use nonverbal communications such as gestures, facial expressions, and eye contact.

While autistic spectrum disorder consists of a broad range of conditions, to make things easier, from here on I will use the term *autism* to refer to autistic spectrum disorder.

#### AUTISM—A MYSTERY

Autism is often associated with children because clear symptoms of autism have to have been displayed by age three in order to get a diagnoses (even if autism stays with you throughout life). There are around sixty million people with autism in the world. In the United States, around 1 in 59 children are diagnosed with autism; in Sweden, around 91,000 people live with autism, and each year around 450 children are diagnosed. The disorder is more common in boys, who are diagnosed four times more than girls.

What causes autism, and why is in on the increase? Studies have shown that heredity plays a large part in autism, such as a Swedish study that attributed 50 percent to hereditary factors. Apart from genetics, researchers have also looked at disruption in the immune system, inflammation, and environmental toxins. In recent years, many studies have appeared that bring gut bacteria to the forefront as one of the hottest candidates to crack the autism code.

#### THE BRIEF GUT-BRAIN WINDOW

Gut flora is established during the first three years of life before it is "grown up." What's also interesting is symptoms of autism appear during the period up until three years of age—it is during these years that the brain development of children with autism start to drastically differ, with some parts growing quicker and others developing more slowly. In other words, the window when gut flora is established coincides with the period when autism develops. Today, researchers agree that gut flora is a deciding factor in the development of the brain, so even if heredity has dominated as an explanation as to why autism occurs, more researchers have started to suspect that the development of gut flora during the first three years may also play a significant role. Most telling is the experiment with sterile mice who grew up devoid of gut flora—their brains shrunk and displayed abnormal development. The mice's behavior was reminiscent of the antisocial behavior of people with autism, and listen to this: when the sterile mice were moved to a normal environment filled with bacteria and other mice that were raised normally, the first group mice's antisocial behavior returned to normal. Researchers believe this was due to "spontaneous transplantation," which is an eloquent way of saying that they had eaten the other mice's feces.

#### IS AUTISM A DISTURBANCE OF THE GUT-BRAIN?

An important lead in the autism mystery is that it is well-known that autism is often related to stomach and gut problems. Typical issues are gassiness, diarrhea, stomachache, and constipation, with the latter being a common symptom in children with autism (85 percent). Stomach and gut problems are so common among people with autism that they are classed as a comorbid symptom of autism (comorbidity means several diagnoses in a patient at the same time). This explains why more scientists believe that disruption in the dialogue between the gut and brain are related to autism.

If there was a lack of interest a few years ago, the amount of studies looking at the link between autism and gut flora has exploded lately. What do these studies reveal? First, they show a clear link between an abnormal gut flora and brain development that deviates from the norm, which autism involves. Second, a variety of studies show that the gut flora in people with autism clearly differs from those in others. Third, and perhaps most interesting, preliminary research shows that treatment that improves gut flora has even improved symptoms of autism. This discovery has already made its way into international news and given hope to parents of children with autism.

#### THE MOTHER'S LIFESTYLE MATTERS

There is much to think about for a mother-to-be. It seems to be the case that a mother's diet and state of health during a pregnancy can affect her child's future health. Animal studies have shown that a diet high in saturated fats during pregnancy lowers the level of good bacteria in the gut of the offspring, which has shown to trigger autism-type symptoms. Perhaps this could be the case for humans, too. So even if the LCHF trend has pushed the notion that food with a high fat content s okay for us, it seems sensible to avoid foods containing saturated fats (but not omega-3) especially during pregnancy. And it is not enough to keep an eye on the food you eat; research indicates that pregnant women who suffer from diabetes and/or obesity are more likely to some extent to have children with autism. It is important during pregnancy to look after your health and gut flora by minimizing stress and living as healthily as you can.

#### THE IMPORTANCE OF GIVING BIRTH VAGINALLY AND BREASTFEEDING

It is known that the risk of autism is higher in children born by means of  cesarean sections compared to those born vaginally. So far no one really knows why, but more scientists are starting to believe that it must have something to do with the fact that children born by cesareans do not get enough beneficial bacteria in their mother's birth canal. While the gut flora in children who are born vaginally is reminiscent of their mother's vaginal gut flora, which is dominated by beneficial bacteria such as lactobacillus, prevotella, and/or sneathia, the gut flora in children born by cesarean section is dominated by harmful bacteria that can be found on the mother's skin, such as staphylococcus, corynebacterium, and propionibacterium.

You also need to keep an eye on what you feed your baby during the first three years.

Breast milk is recommended over formula since breastfeeding has been linked to a normal development of the baby's brain. Babies who are given formula have been shown to have a worse gut flora, which has been linked to a higher rate of autism. But if the child is breastfed for more than six months, there is a reduced risk of developing autism. Breastmilk contains several probiotic bacteria and even the prebiotic GOS (see p. 93). These days, many food producers add GOS and beneficial bacteria to formula. Other factors that affect a child's gut flora are stress (even after pregnancy), the child's diet, and their environment.

Even if gut bacteria appear to have a role in the risk of developing autism in children, we can't forget that heredity also plays a deciding factor (50 percent).

#### POO TRANSPLANTS REDUCE AUTISM SYMPTOMS

Fecal transplants, that is, transplanting feces from one person to another, has now been used in trials in children with autism. You first cleanse out the sick gut flora using antibiotics and then introduce a healthy gut flora from a donor. In a noted study from 2017, children with autism between ages seven and seventeen with unhealthy gut flora took antibiotics for fourteen days, which was followed by twelve to twenty-four hours of fasting and gut cleansing, and then their gut flora was repopulated with a high dose of gut flora from a "normal" person. They were then asked to maintain their new gut flora with lower doses of probiotic bacteria for seven to eight weeks. An analysis of the children's gut flora after eight weeks revealed that the introduction of healthy gut flora had been successful, with positive changes in the autistic children's gut flora. Diversity had increased, and the amount of good bacteria like bifidobacterium, prevotella, and desulfovibrio had also increased. Further results showed that the stomach and gut problems in these children (constipation, diarrhea, stomachaches, and so on) drastically reduced by 80 percent, remaining for eight weeks after the treatment. In a similar way, typical autistic behaviors and symptoms also improved over the eight weeks after the treatment. This study shows that in order to maintain their newly gained gut-brain health, the children would need a supplement of living probiotic bacteria every eight weeks. Even if larger placebo-controlled studies are needed before fecal transplantations can be used as a treatment for autism, scientific advances such as these are encouraging to all parents who have children with autism, especially in light of the fact that there are currently no effective treatments to reduce symptoms.

#### PROBIOTICS: LACTIC ACID BACTERIA AND SYMPTOMS OF AUTISM

As new research shows that fecal transplants can reduce autism symptoms in children, another question is whether lactic acid bacteria ingested via food or as a supplement can also work on serious neuropsychiatric disorders like autism. The answer seems to be yes! Early studies show that regular lactic acid bacteria can normalize gut flora, strengthen the mucous membrane, and improve autism-like symptoms, such as antisocial behavior and stomach and gut problems. This is fantastic news, but since few studies have been placebo-controlled, we have to interpret the results with caution.

The exact mix of bacteria has varied between studies. Usually a variety of classic lactic acid bacteria has been used (bifidobacterium and lactobacillus), which can be found in fermented foods like yogurt and kimchi. Among the reported effects, the following are worth mentioning: reduction of the malignant species Clostridium, better gut function, reduced anxiety, reduced antisocial behavior and reduced communication difficulties, increased ability to concentrate and to follow directions, etc. In an interesting case, a boy with severe autism took a probiotic cocktail consisting of ten beneficial bacteria over four weeks. Despite the short treatment time and the boy's serious condition, both his stomach and gut problems were improved as well as other symptoms typical of autism. Even if larger and better placebo-controlled studies are needed, initial studies show that gut flora and autism seem to be closely connected.

#### ANTIBIOTICS ARE GOOD AND BAD

Research shows that children who are treated with antibiotics during their first three years have a significantly lower diversity of gut bacteria. This is not exactly news as we know that antibiotics knock out both good and bad bacteria.

Since diversity is a sign of a healthy gut flora and a good prerequisite for a strong immune system and brain health, it's not good news for children who are being treated with too many unnecessary antibiotics. Remember—a human's gut flora establishes during the first three years, a critical period where the development of gut flora goes hand in hand with the development of the brain. A large population-based study showed that the mother's intake of antibiotics during pregnancy worsens the gut flora in newborns, which in turn increases the risk of autism in children. However, antibiotics don't always give negative side effects; they have also been shown to improve stomach and gut problems (like diarrhea) and autistic behavior (even if just during a brief period), which is probably because the antibiotics have knocked out disease-promoting bacteria. In other words, antibiotics are neither good or bad, even in the context of autism. (See p. 65 about Alzheimer's and antibiotics.) The main message here is that the composition of gut bacteria appears to play a central role in autism, where manipulation of gut flora is able to regulate autism symptoms.

### ADHD and gut bacteria

ADHD is the world's most common neuropsychiatric diagnosis, which normally begins during schooling age. Of all children diagnosed with ADHD, around 30 to 50 percent retain this diagnosis as a grown-up. In 2016, 6.1 million children in the United States were diagnosed with ADHD (approximately 9.4 percent of the population); in Sweden, around 64,000 people have ADHD, and 2,800 new cases are diagnosed every year, mostly in boys. The amount of people who have been diagnosed with ADHD has drastically increased over the past few years. Many believe this is not really about an increase, and rather about newly discovered ways of diagnosing cases that would have previously slipped through the net. Others feel that the increase is too high to just be attributed to new diagnostic methods. There are also those who suggest that ADHD is a neurological profile and not a disorder, and that people with ADHD just don't fit with our modern and mainly sedentary society. This is why ADHD is often considered a personality trait and social construction rather than a disorder.

#### A DISTURBANCE OF DOPAMINE AND OTHER NEUROTRASMITTERS

What is ADHD? It stands for *attention-deficit/hyperactivity disorder* and is characterized by three core symptoms: inattention, impulsivity, and hyperactivity. Difficulty in concentration in children with ADHD can lead to learning problems, bad school results, and even disturbing and aggressive behaviors. The underlying cause of ADHD is usually unknown, even if ADHD has also been shown to have high heredity, just like autism. Above all, ADHD has been linked to disturbances in dopamine and noradrenaline, which are important for concentration, attention, and impulse control. Scientists have seen that the genes controlling these neurotransmitters in the brain are different in people with ADHD. When it comes to the link to gut flora, research is scant compared to the vast amount of studies on autism and gut bacteria. However, research is moving so fast that it won't be long until we will know more.

#### CAN THE ANSWER TO THE ADHD PUZZLE BE FOUND IN THE GUT?

Similar to autism, ADHD goes hand in hand with stomach and gut problems and increased inflammation in the blood, and most people with ADHD also suffer stomach and gut problems, which makes the psychiatric suffering worse. A huge study that looked at 742,939 children showed that those with ADHD had much higher instances of constipation than those without. As we know, a stomach that is not working well, as well as an imbalance in gut flora, makes the body and brain more inflamed. Studies also show that inflammatory products in the blood are more common in children with ADHD than those without.

#### CAN PROBIOTICS PREVENT ADHD?

As I've mentioned, there are hardly any clinical studies looking at gut flora's role in ADHD at the moment. Therefore, a small study from Finland has been given a disproportionate amount of attention. The study, published in 2016, was conducted on seventy-five newborns, where some were treated with a probiotic containing the lactic acid bacteria *L. rhamnosus* and others were given a placebo. Researchers waited thirteen years to follow these children as they grew up. The results were that none of the children who received probiotics had a diagnosis of ADHD or Asperger's. However, 17 percent (six out of thirty-five) of the children who had been given a placebo had ADHD or Asperger's. Researchers drew the conclusion that a newborn's ingestion of probiotic lactic acid bacteria can reduce the risk of developing ADHD or Asperger's—though no one really knows at the moment how convincing this is. But even if it was a small study, it has encouraged other researchers to further study the link between ADHD and gut bacteria in Sweden and the Netherlands, among other places.

#### CAN ANTIBIOTICS INCREASE THE RISK FOR ADHD?

Currently, a study is being conducted on ADHD at the Karolinska Institute in Sweden that examines the link between the brain and gut.

**Soki Choi reflects on neurological diversity**

Diversity rewards itself: the earth prefers to thrive with many species of organisms, humans fare better by eating various plants and animals, bacterial diversity in the gut is better for your body and brain, and so on. Despite this universal wisdom, humans have stupidly done their best to make animals, plants, bacteria, and even other humans extinct in our brutal approach to make it to the top of the food pyramid. When will we learn that our predatory tendencies of driving other species to extinction will only harm ourselves? In the same way that bacterial diversity is beneficial, I am convinced that neurological diversity pays as well. Which is why I find it deeply problematic that ADHD and autism are described with negative words such as *disorder* or *impairment* (even if it might make sense in severe autism, for example). Talking about ADHD and autism in negative terms is especially strange when it is said that everyone is on the ADHD spectrum. The spectrums for both ADHD and autistic spectrum disorder are broad, and geniuses like Michelangelo, Newton, Darwin, and Einstein were thought to be high-functioning in some form of autistic spectrum disorder (the diagnosis did not exist in those days). This is why I like to look at neuropsychiatric disorders as neurological profiles or personality traits rather than use terms like *disease*. People with ADHD who are born into modern times might just not fit into our sedentary lifestyles.

First, researchers are looking into whether antibiotics in the first years after birth increases the risk of ADHD. We know that the gut flora in young children is especially sensitive to stress. Overuse of antibiotics can harm the gut flora, which, hypothetically, can contribute to ADHD. Second, researchers are investigating whether inflammation-promoting bacterial products pass through the gut and into the bloodstream in children with ADHD, since we know that inflammatory products are more common in children with ADHD. Third, researchers are investigating whether a better gut flora increases well-being in children with ADHD and whether this is because bacteria affect the immune system.

A leading Swedish scientist Catharina Lavebratt may have an answer to the question of whether bad gut flora can cause ADHD. She believes that despite not knowing enough to conclusively say that a bad gut flora causes ADHD, it could be the case that a strong gut flora is a protective factor for genetic predisposition for ADHD. As we have seen, autism symptoms are greatly improved with probiotics. Lavebratt doesn't believe that ADHD symptoms can disappear but that probiotics can ease ADHD via a better gut system and improved psychiatric symptoms. Essentially, she believes that probiotics can be used to complement other treatments for ADHD.

#### PEOPLE WITH ADHD HAVE A DIFFERENT GUT FLORA

A Dutch study published in September 2017 was the first to describe the composition of gut flora in young people and adults with ADHD. Researchers found that patients with ADHD had a different composition of gut bacteria when compared to a control group. Even if the exact mechanisms behind ADHD are still not clear, researchers believe that this different gut flora could cause disturbances in dopamine production, which in turn hampers the reward response. Despite the fact that we need more and larger studies, this first study points to the notion that gut flora has a part to play in the ADHD mystery.

### Promising Research

In light of the fact that researchers have previously been stumbling in the dark for clues, the link between gut flora and neuropsychiatric diagnoses like autism and ADHD is a breakthrough. As we've seen, preliminary research has shown a clear correlation between neuropsychiatric symptoms and difficult gut problems. Some researchers even suspect causation.

It is with great interest and suspense that we follow this promising research on the role of gut bacteria in these diagnoses.

Simply put, groundbreaking research is revolutionizing our view and treatment of mental health disorders (stress, anxiety, and depression), age-related diseases (Alzheimer's and Parkinson's), and neuropsychiatric diagnoses (autism and ADHD)—all common diagnoses relating to the brain.

# *A summary of chapter 3*

**The role of gut bacteria in stress, anxiety, and depression**

• Stress fuels harmful gut bacteria and also contributes to a leaky gut.

• Inflammation in the body can permeate into the brain.

• Depression can be inflammation in the brain (neuroinflammation).

• Lactic acid bacteria can reduce stress, anxiety, and depression.

• Fiber (GOS) has been shown to reduce anxiety and depression.

• Food with large amounts of saturated fats and sugar contribute to inflammation in the brain.

**The role of gut bacteria in Alzheimer's and Parkinson's**

• Gut flora is thought to be an important factor in driving Alzheimer's and Parkinson's.

• Patients with Alzheimer's have a lower bacterial diversity and an inflammation-promoting gut flora.

• Probiotics can reduce "Alzheimer's" plaque in the brain.

• Antibiotics can change gut flora so that "Alzheimer's" plaque is reduced.

• The gut flora in patients with Parkinson's is teeming with harmful bacteria.

• Parkinson's is believed to start in the gut since "Parkinson's" plaque has been discovered in the gut.

**The role of gut bacteria in autism and ADHD**

• Gut flora plays a central role in autism.

• The gut flora in people with autism is clearly different from that in others.

• People with autism often have stomach and gut problems.

• A mother's lifestyle during pregnancy, the birthing method, and how the baby is fed during their first years influence the risk of autism.

• New, healthy gut flora via poo donations reduced autism symptoms in children.

CHAPTER 4

# Let food be your medicine

## *Food takes to the medical stage*

In our overfed society, quality of life is no longer just about life span but also how we can increase the number of healthy years we live—health span. The acceleration of chronic diseases and mental health problems in the West reveal that something has gone very wrong in our quest for material wealth and a long and healthy life.

We can find hope in the relatively new discovery of the existence of bacterial intelligence in our guts. Who would have thought that way down in our guts we would have our own pharmaceutical factory where trillions of bacteria act as our very own mini-doctors? Depending on what we feed our mini-doctors, they'll give us anything from anti-inflammatory butyric acid to antidepressant feel-good molecules—without the side effects. And the wonderful thing is that we are able to influence our own gut flora and brain. Our gut flora and the brain's plasticity are constantly changing, reflecting what we feed them with—our food and thoughts.

We now also know that the gut and brain are intimately connected in what scientists call the gut-brain axis, and the dialogue goes both ways. If you feed your brain with stressful thoughts, your gut flora is negatively affected; and if you feed your gut flora with bad food, your brain is negatively affected.

That food plays a decisive role in your health is not news. The father of medicine, Hippocrates, stated twenty-five hundred years ago: "Let food be your medicine and medicine your food." Despite his wisdom, diet was most recently kept away at arm's length by Western doctors—until now. As you have seen in previous chapters, increasing evidence shows that fiber (prebiotics) and bacteria (probiotics) in food don't just play a preventative role as a lifestyle medicine; they also have the potential to treat more severe ailments such as depression, Alzheimer's, and autism. Many researchers and doctors believe that food will, in all seriousness, join the medical arena very soon.

So, which foods top the list of probiotics? The answer is kombucha and kimchi, which are both stuffed with healthy fiber and bacteria. But you'll have to wait for the next chapter to find out more about them; first, we are going to go on a journey where I'll take you through four historic revolutions that, in different ways, have accidentally "offended" the bacterial intelligence in our gut throughout evolution. Let's dive straight into the psychobiotic world of food, and prepare to get plenty of tips on how to regulate your gut flora using food in order to protect and strengthen your brain.

## *Historical offenses against our gut flora*

As we know, bacteria laid the evolutionary foundation for plants, animals, and humans; compared to bacteria, humans are evolutionary newbies. Since then, our hardworking bacteria have lived side by side with humans in perfect harmony. Our hunting forebears are believed to have walked roughly ten kilometers every day, forced to fast now and again, and eaten a varied diet consisting of hundreds of plants

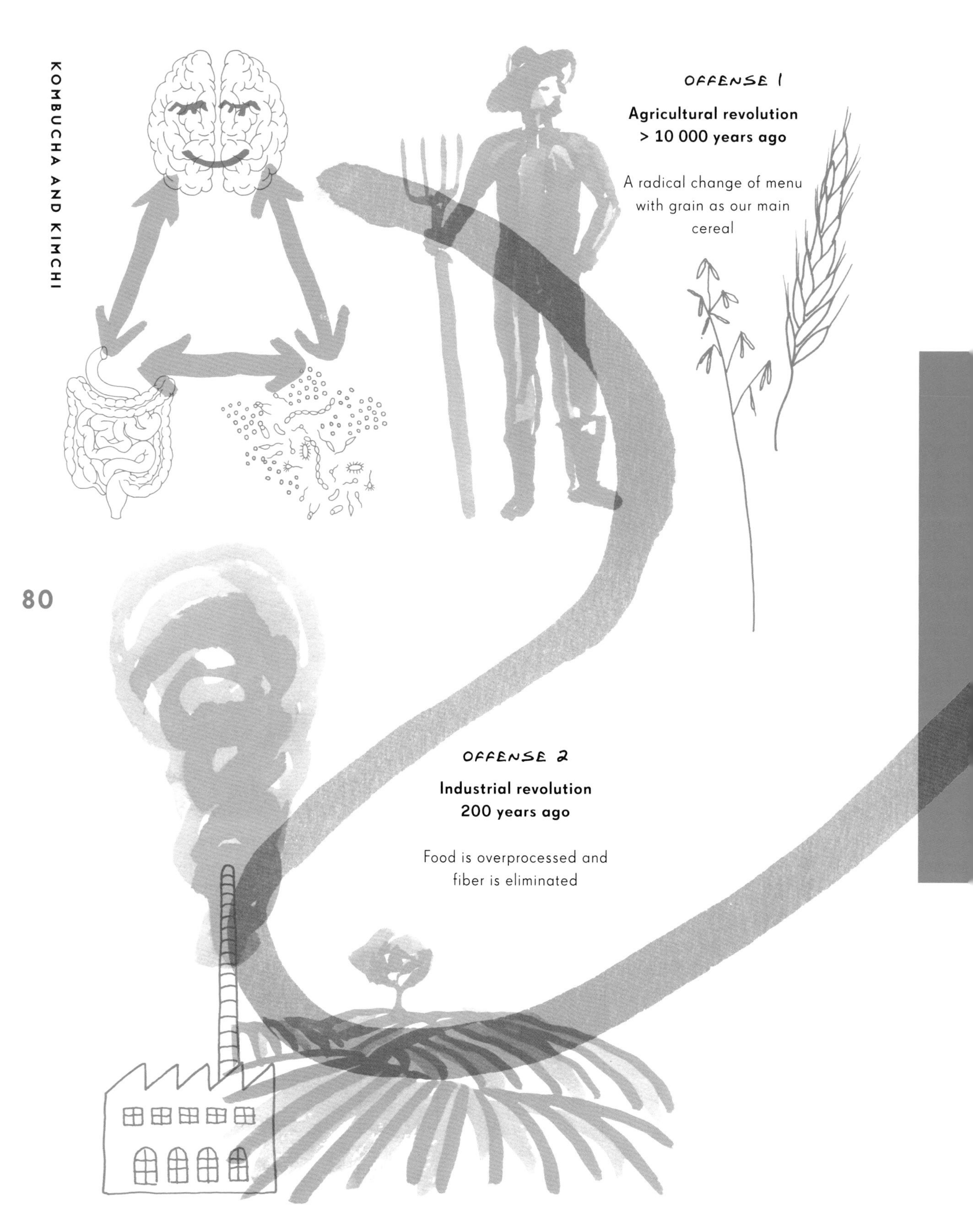
OFFENSE 1
Agricultural revolution
> 10 000 years ago
A radical change of menu with grain as our main cereal
OFFENSE 2
Industrial revolution
200 years ago
Food is overprocessed and fiber is eliminated

OFFENSE 3

**The antibiotic revolution from the 1950s onward**

Antibiotics take care of our infections but deplete our gut flora



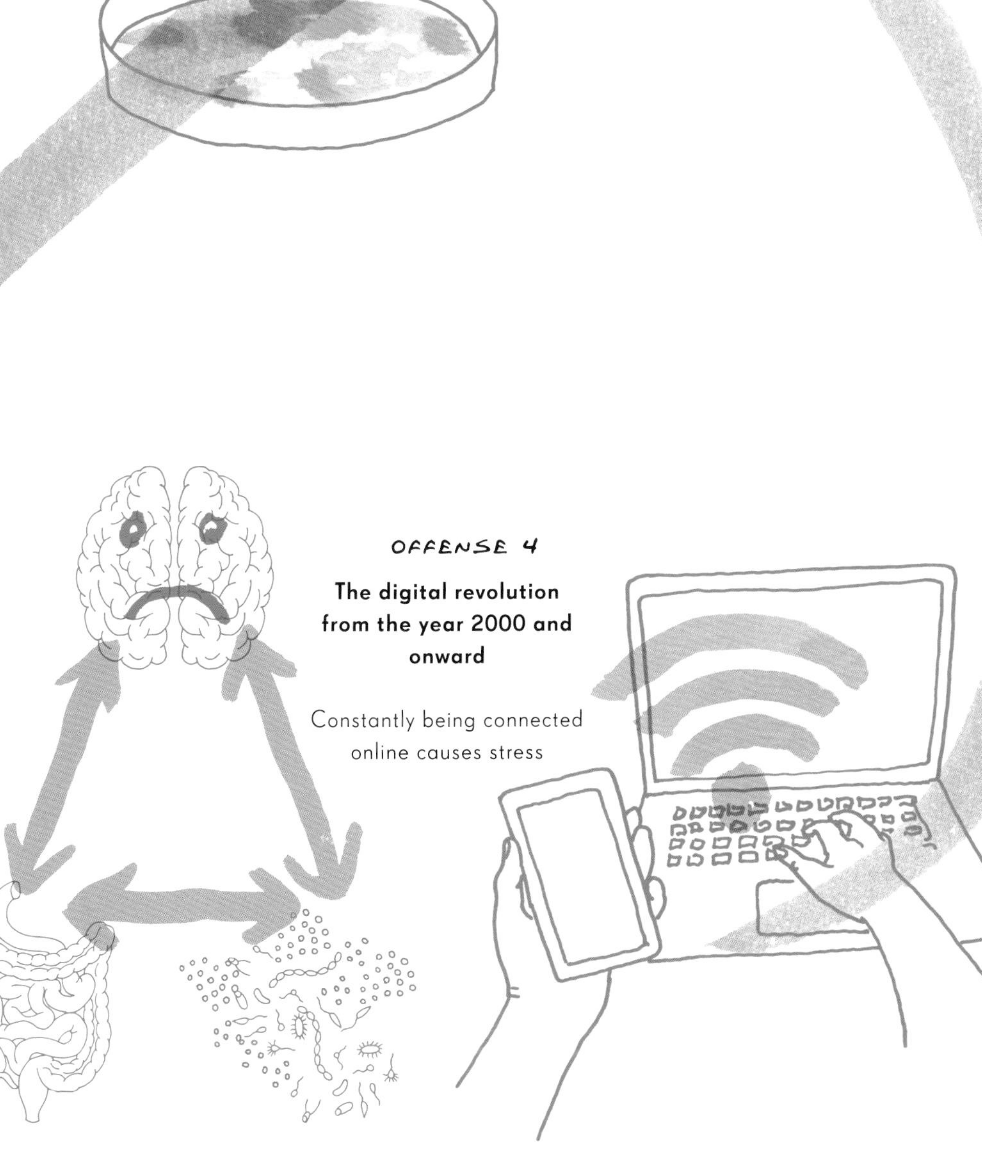

OFFENSE 4

**The digital revolution from the year 2000 and onward**

Constantly being connected online causes stress

and animals. All this made our bacteria happy, and they helped to protect us against obesity, diabetes, cancer, and cardiovascular disease. Our symbiotic contract with bacteria was successful and lasted several millions of years. One day, around ten thousand years ago, everything changed. The agricultural revolution began, which was the beginning of a host of biological offenses against our bacterial friends, something we are still suffering from today. To get a deeper understanding of how and why our gut flora has been so radically depleted in only ten thousand years, I will take you on a historical odyssey that looks at four revolutions that have offended our gut flora in different ways. They are:

1) The agricultural revolution
2) The industrial revolution
3) The antibiotic revolution
4) The ongoing digital revolution

Each revolution is considered to have brought big gains for humankind, such as medicine, population increase, longer life span, and new technology. However, we can't ignore that progress has come at a high price in the form of the current ill-health in our societies, which is spreading like an epidemic across the modern world. Our acceleration of the chase for artificial intelligence high up in the clouds has, along the way, caused us to lose our bacterial intelligence deep inside our bodies.



OFFENSE 1

## The agricultural revolution—a radical menu change

For 2.5 million years, our forebears survived by picking berries and fruit and hunting wild animals. Our symbiotic contract with bacteria was handled well with a rich diversity of gut flora that was reflected in our hunter-gatherer diet of plants and animals.

However, ten thousand years ago, something occurred: the agricultural revolution. Humans started to spend most of their time looking after a handful of animals and plant types as we became static farmers. With the agricultural revolution, our varied menu of yesteryear started to change radically, leading to over 50 percent of all calories coming from a handful of grains such as wheat, oat, rice, corn, and rye—a diet that still sustains humans today. If you think about it, a day seldom passes where you don't eat any one of these grains. From the hundreds of species that our forebears hunted and gathered, the agricultural revolution reduced our diet to just a few elements. The result has been a drastic depletion of the gut flora of the modern human.

From a biological perspective, ten thousand years occur in the blink of an eye, equivalent to only 1 percent of humankind's total history, which means that we are almost genetically identical to our forebears who lived before the agricultural revolution. And while our boost in calorie intake did of course increase our total amount of food as well as lead to population growth and a longer life span, in exchange we now eat a much less varied diet and have a drastically reduced variety of gut bacterial species. Our dependence on a small amount of cultivated crops has completely depleted our gut flora. If our current epidemic of "unexplained" chronic Western diseases could to a large extent be blamed on depleted gut flora (which recent research points to), then we can trace the root cause all the way back to the agricultural revolution. While the agricultural revolution was a big leap forward for humankind that freed up our time for art, music, inventions, and so on, in hindsight we can agree that we've had to pay a high price in the form of today's chronic diseases and mental health problems, which are spreading like an unstoppable plague.

#### OUR INVALUABLE WINDOW TO THE PAST

With groundbreaking discovery of gut flora's pivotal role to our health and brain, a serious chase is now ongoing to figure out how to enrich our gut flora. To uncover all the clues on how we can diversify our gut flora, research into modern-day's remaining hunter-gatherer tribes gives us an invaluable window to the past. These people still live as our forebears did ten thousand years ago, and ironically enough the search for the West's "Holy Grail"— a long, healthy life—has led researchers to those parts of the world that are considered the "poorest" on paper, economically speaking. In terms of the richness of variety in their gut flora and other health parameters, these subjects beat their counterparts in "richer" countries, hands down. So the question is: who is richer?

The lifestyles and gut flora of the Yanomami tribe in the Amazon and the Hadza people in Tanzania have been studied recently by enthusiastic scientists. The two tribes hunt and collect plants according to the season and have little or no access to modern processed foods, medicine, antibiotics, or hygiene articles. In addition, both tribes have a huge diversity of bacteria in their gut flora compared to Western people. Let's take a closer look at what the Yanomami tribe eat.

Yanomami live in one of the most remote parts of the Amazon by the border between Brazil and Venezuela. Their diet is based on cooked bananas, cassava, vegetables, fruits, and insects. Along with that, they also eat hundreds of different plants, berries, and seeds, both as food and for medicinal purposes. In addition, they make use of fermentation in their food, which contributes living bacteria to their diet. Sometimes they eat animal products like fish, birds, frogs, beetles, larvae, peccary. and monkeys, but it is far from the amount consumed in the West. The meat is also wild and lean. When two unconnected research teams were given permission to test their stool samples, the results were striking. First, the Yanomami people had a huge variety of bacteria in their gut flora when compared to Westerners. Second, many bacterial species were unique to just the Yanomami people, and tests showed no evidence of obesity. In addition, the Yanomami people had among the lowest blood lipids that had ever been measured on people. They had no diabetes, high blood pressure, cardiovascular diseases, or autoimmune diseases.

For most Westerners it is slightly unrealistic and not very appealing to return to the life that our hunter-gatherer forebears led. The risk of dying from injuries from wild predators or wars between tribes is larger, which is why life expectancy is a lot higher in the modern world. From a bacterial perspective, however, we have a lot to learn from the few hunter-gatherer tribes that remain. It is clear that they have a much richer and more varied gut flora, which goes hand in hand with the health benefits they have that we in the West can only dream about.

In hindsight, we can concede that modern humans with their depleted gut flora have broken their symbiotic contract with bacteria that evolution once created a long time ago.

Even today, the food industry is dominated by production methods that do not take into account the health of our gut flora.

OFFENSE 2

## The overprocessed food of the industrial revolution

The industrial revolution's offense against our gut flora can be summarized as this: processed, artificial food with too much sugar, i.e., low-quality food. Processed food (finely ground wheat flour, fruit juices, etc.) can be found on shelves everywhere and are devoid of important fiber that acts as nourishment for our good bacteria. Artificial food with plenty of additives are also widely available, and sugar in all its forms have crept in just about everywhere. All you have to do is look at food labels to see a long list of chemical additives that prolong the sell-by date, heighten taste and flavor, or soften the food. Many of these additives have been shown to have a devastating effect on our gut flora.

Those of us who live in the West eat a lot of processed, calorie-rich, and nutrient-poor food, meaning that we often don't get enough fiber in our diet; however, we do get too many harmful additives. The introduction of processed foods into our daily lives can be traced back to the end of the nineteenth century when the food industry was looking for ways to reduce fiber in food. Take wheat flour for example: industrial mills were consciously designed to remove bran and wheat germ from grain so that flour could be milled as finely as possible. Refined wheat flour was used to make attractive and tasty breads and cakes. White flour became a success and no one considered the reality that the fiber was now missing.

Even today, the food industry is dominated by production methods that do not take into account the health of our gut flora and work against our biological intelligence. The production of processed food like white bread, sugar, and orange juice most likely didn't begin with harmful intentions, but once the market was established, both producers and consumers were unwilling to change their behaviors and structures. Instead, we have seen a huge growth in the commercial market for pharmaceuticals in response to diet-related health problems that the processed food industry has caused. Even if it is tempting to point the finger at large food and pharmaceutical companies, I somewhat reluctantly agree that consumers also bear a responsibility—despite widespread knowledge and information that is at our fingertips, we continue to buy and consume foods that harm our health. Ultimately, the logic of industry is to sell what consumers buy, so the more organic, fiber-rich foods we buy, for example, the more growers and producers of said foods will benefit and be incentivized. In addition, the food industry is also starting to add prebiotic fiber such as inulin and oligofructose into food. Here's to hoping that the food industry will continue to reduce the historical offenses made against our gut flora and mental health that the elimination of fiber from our diet has caused. In the meantime, consumers need to stimulate the industry by actively and consistently choosing natural, organic foods that benefit our gut flora and mental health.

#### THE RISE AND FALL OF MCDONALD'S

Did you know that once upon a time McDonald's had a large part to play in the emancipation of women from the kitchen? Suddenly, the whole family could eat out for a small sum, which is considered to have helped relieve women's cooking duties in the kitchen. Today, in light of the well-known harmful effects of a McDonald's diet on our health, in seems unbelievable that McDonald's was once so unquestionably popular. Well-documented studies show that the McDonald's diet, or SAD (also known as the *standard American diet*), doesn't just lead to diabetes and obesity, but also to mental health problems. The standard American diet is highly processed with a high sugar count, high amount of saturated fats, too few nutrients, too little fiber, and no good bacteria. Think ground meat (sausages and hamburgers), sweet foods (soda, ice cream, sweets, jam, and juice), salty snacks (chips, cheese puffs) and wheat flour (white bread, biscuits, pancakes, cakes).

Did you know that if you eat a hot dog or a bacon sandwich every day, you reduce your life span by two years? Several large studies, including a Norwegian study with twenty-three thousand participants, showed that a standard American diet also led to depression and anxiety. Junk food can harm the critical blood-brain barrier, among other things, making it possible for harmful toxins to reach your brain. So, if you want to replace harmful bacteria that thrive on a McDonald's diet and avoid feeding an unhealthy gut flora, it is vital to stop eating junk food—end of story. Soon, I'll show you what you should be eating instead.

OFFENSE 3

## The antibiotic revolution brings on mass extinction

In 1928, the Scotsman Sir Alexander Fleming discovered antibiotics by accident. It happened when he had left a bacterial culture sitting out in a rush to go on vacation. He had no idea that his discovery on his return—that a fungus had contaminated the culture and destroyed the bacteria—would revolutionize the medical world. There's no doubt that antibiotics have saved, and continues to save, millions of people's lives every year. Most of us have probably suffered from and been cured of a normal infection that, in the past without antibiotics, might have taken our lives. In addition, antibiotics are thought to add ten years to the average life span. The discovery of antibiotics was so big that researchers and doctors believed that antibiotics would lead to the end of all human infections within twenty years.

This belief in the superpower of antibiotics led to a mass production during World War II, and since then they have been consumed like candy around the world, especially in the United States. In the United States alone, around 250 million courses of antibiotics are prescribed each year, while credit goes to Sweden and Denmark for being the most restrictive countries, both prescribing only half the antibiotics per capita compared to the United States. Sweden and Denmark also use a larger variety of antibiotics with a narrower spectrum, which allows for more accurate treatment and causes less harm to gut flora.

Many of us may know that a large threat is caused by multiresistant bacteria—bacteria that are resilient against antibiotics—which makes it difficult or impossible for doctors to treat diseases caused by these bacteria. Multiresistant bacteria were discovered almost immediately after the first large-scale use of penicillin in the 1940s, and they still wage their war today. Each year, multiresistant bacteria claim seven hundred thousand lives. If the spread and speed of this epidemic is not stopped, it is estimated that ten million people will die from multiresistant bacteria in 2050.

Antibiotics have infiltrated all aspects of our society, from water reservoirs to the food chain (found in meat, fish, and vegetables). It is impossible to avoid regular microdoses of antibiotics—whether you want to or not. Above all, the use of antibiotics has weakened our gut flora. More and more researchers suspect that the unexplained increase of chronic Western illnesses has been driven by the widespread use of antibiotics, which, together with our Western lifestyle, have depleted our gut flora.

New studies also show that antibiotics can lead to a reduced brain capacity as well as an increase in depressive behavior in animals. Antibiotics reduce the creation of brain cells in the hippocampus, which is a structure in the brain that is important for memory and emotional regulation. Research also shows that a child who has been treated with antibiotics in the first three years of life has a great deal less varied gut flora. This is worrying, since variety is, as I've mentioned, an indication of a healthy gut flora, and it gives a better health prognosis, including good mental health.

#### A FEW GOOD TIPS WHEN TAKING ANTIBIOTICS

If you and your child have to take antibiotics, here's some good advice to follow:

1) **Ask for a narrow-spectrum antibiotic:** Often, a doctor will prescribe antibiotics with a broad spectrum since it is easier. This is almost like removing an organ as a

wide-spectrum antibiotic knocks out your entire gut flora, including the beneficial bacteria (the exception, of course, are dangerous multiresistant bacteria that can make you seriously ill and that are able to resist the drug). In addition, it can take months, even years, to restore your gut flora after treatment with a broad-spectrum antibiotic.

2) **Ask for a procalcitonin test:** Antibiotics work on bacteria but not on viruses and colds, and things like throat infections are often caused by a virus that antibiotics won't work on. Confirm that your doctor has done a procalcitonin test to see if your infection is due to bacteria or a virus.

3) **Compensate with probiotics:** if you have to take antibiotics, make sure you supplement your treatment regularly with beneficial bacteria, which means taking probiotics to compensate for the antibiotics' attack on good bacteria. Good bacteria can be found in tangy, fermented foods like yogurt, kimchi, and kombucha or as a supplement. Mostly, different species from the *Lactobacillus* genus can help to replenish your depleted gut flora with helpful bacteria. Even prebiotics in the form of fiber are good to eat during this time as they act as food to the probiotic bacteria.

#### THE POSITIVE FUTURE ROLE OF ANTIBIOTICS

Even if research shows that antibiotics generally have a negative effect on our gut flora, they may actually play a more positive role in the future. Many studies show that antibiotics can knock out harmful bacteria that contribute to anxiety, depression, Alzheimer's, and autism. Researchers around the world are already hard at work trying to pair bacteria with various diagnoses in the hopes of soon being able to use narrow-spectrum and accurate antibiotic treatment to only knock out illness-inducing bacteria without harming good bacteria. It would be a huge medical breakthrough if antibiotics were to become a part of the future treatment for depression and Alzheimer's.

OFFENSE 4

## Stress and the digital revolution

Apart from food and antibiotics, stress is a powerful way to offend your gut flora. In 2017, the American Psychological Association's annual survey on stress reported the most significant increase in stress in their ten-year history, with stress levels rising to a high of 5.1 on a scale from one to ten. Meanwhile, the amount of people in Sweden who suffer from serious stress symptoms has increased by over 100 percent in just ten years from 2006 to 2016. Apart from stress, in this digital age the use of medication for ADHD for problems with concentration and attention has increased over the past ten years among adults who don't even have ADHD. During this same period, the use of antidepressants has doubled among young people. Similar developments can be seen in other countries, and whatever numbers we look at, we can't avoid the fact that the drastic increase of mental health problems and psychopharmaceuticals coincide with our current digital revolution.

Our brain is bombarded by a digital stream of information twenty-four hours a day, and smartphones, iPads, computers, and apps constantly attract our attention. Just as no one in the 1950s could have predicted the devastating health effects that a McDonald's diet and antibiotics would have decades later, we, too, don't know the long-term harm that this digital experiment will bring. All we know is that we're now finding ourselves in the middle of a digitally dominated society that will bring about certain future consequences to the health of our gut and brain. Research on the influence of the digital revolution is starting to trickle in, and we can take a look at what recent studies have discovered about the negative effects of digital media on our gut flora and mental health.

#### A DIGITAL LIFE

In the United States, one in three babies start to use digital media before they can talk. American teenagers spend nine hours a day on social media, and two out of three teens do their homework while simultaneously chatting with friends. In Sweden, millennials devote nearly four hours a day to social media and use their mobile phone roughly every second minute. Among office workers, 45 percent of time goes to emailing and phone calls, which they perceive as stressful. In addition, half of all Swedes check their work email while on vacation and use the Internet to work in their free time. Five of the six biggest sources of workplace stress are digital: a high expectation of being accessible, technical developments, information overload, always being online, and being surpassed by new digital talents and trends. In other words, the digital world has overtaken our lives.

#### ILL DIGITAL HEALTH

What effect does our increasingly widespread digital life have on our mental health? New studies show that the longer you sit at a computer or with a smartphone, the lower your well-being; the more you use social media, the more depressed you'll feel; the more selfies you look at, the lower your self-esteem and life satisfaction; the more status updates on Facebook, the worse you feel; and so on.

Research shows that depression and anxiety are as much as three times more common among people who use many different forms of social media compared to those who use fewer or none. People who multitask are more easily distracted, have a worse memory, and a worse attention span. A frequent use of smartphones also goes hand in hand with lower impulse control (which could partially explain the increased use of ADHD medication). The light from mobile phones has also been shown to affect our circadian rhythm by affecting the sleep hormone melatonin. It's not surprising that people who use a lot of social media have been shown to have two to three times the amount of sleep problems compared to others.

#### DIGITAL HEROIN

More parents are also reporting aggressive behaviors in young children when digital screens are removed. Even worse, screens can make children apathetic and uninterested when they are not "plugged in." Studies on brain images have shown that digital screens stimulate the brain in the same way cocaine does, hence the popular term *digital heroin* among researchers. "Likes" on Facebook also activate the same reward system in the brain as food, sex, alcohol, and cigarettes.

Strangely enough, research shows that humans have a harder time resisting the impulse to use social media than alcohol and cigarettes. Changes in certain neural pathways have also been observed in young people who are addicted to mobile phones. The excessive use of social media is becoming more and more related to lower grades in school and relationship problems off-line, which has led to the term *social media disorder*. Dr. Nicholas Kardaras, a well-known psychologist and addiction expert, suggests that it is easier to treat a heroin addict than to treat a Facebook addict.



**Soki Choi reflects on ADHD in a digital world**

Researchers believe that ADHD has always existed and that we are all on the spectrum. That's not unusual in light of the fact that its core symptoms are inattention, impulsivity, and hyperactivity. Who hasn't experienced a lack of concentration or impulse control—especially in these digital times when we are bombarded by impressions and choices? The use of ADHD medication has increased the most among adults who don't have an ADHD diagnosis but who take medication to control concentration and attention problems.

In the media, ADHD and other such acronyms are used left, right, and center, and we like to diagnose ourselves and others. The only positive is that ADHD and other psychiatric diagnoses have become less stigmatized. At the same time, people who actually have an ADHD diagnosis are at risk of not being taken seriously. With smartphones constantly clamoring for our attention, it's not just a wild guess that the prescription of ADHD medication and ADHD diagnoses will continue to rise. The question is how much digital stress our ancient brain can deal with—despite the medicine.

**DIGITAL NEWBIES**

One thing is certain: our brains are not prepared for a digital society. If you look at the history of humanity as a period of twenty-four hours, then we were connected to the Internet at 23.59.50 hours, that is to say one second ago. Even if many people are hailing the benefits of the digital revolution, it is important to remember that this comes at the cost of digital stress, which is detrimental to mental health. There is no doubt that we are currently in the middle of a social experiment.

It is clear that we are sabotaging our gut flora with digital stress.

With the new discovery of the biological supercomputer in our guts, the focus is now on how to minimize the digital damage to our gut flora and brain. How do we balance new artificial intelligence with our ancient biological gut intelligence? How can we stop offending our gut-brain axis with digital stress? Collected research shows that food is probably the best way to protect your gut-brain axis.

## *Eat your way to a stronger brain*

Hippocrates's famous proverb of letting food be our medicine and medicine our food resonates today in an age of growing ill-health. Countless studies have proven that food is one of the best ways to nurture our gut flora. Hippocrates, an early supporter of scientific methods, also said that all illnesses begin in the gut, including mental illness. Few could suspect how right he would be—it would only take 2,500 years for research to finally catch up. It is time to look at how you, with the help of food, can repair the historical offenses against gut flora and boost your brain.

### Psychobiotics take the stage

With hot, new research on gut bacteria's importance to our brain and physiological health, we are guaranteed to hear about prebiotics and probiotics—but what is a psychobiotic? The term *psychobiotic* was coined in 2013 by researchers Ted Dinan and John Cryan as a way to distinguish between bacteria that had a strengthening effect on the brain and our psyche. These bacteria can produce substances that affect the brain (neuroactive) such as serotonin and GABA, and most belong to the genera *Lactobacillus* and *Bifidobacterium*. Psychobiotics have grown to include fiber that stimulates bacteria's production of brain-strengthening substances, and Cryan and Dinan want to go even further to broaden psychobiotics to include all external factors (including exercise and medication) that have a positive effect on our brain and psyche through the regulation of gut flora, though so far at least only fiber and bacteria can be classed as psychobiotics. Let's now look at what types of food are psychobiotic that can strengthen your brain. First, we have prebiotics—or *fiber* as they are known in lay terms.

### Eat more fiber (prebiotics)

We know that fiber is good for the stomach, gut, and even the brain. We should eat at least 30 grams of fiber each day; however, most people in the West barely reach half of that recommendation. *Fiber* is the overall term for complex carbohydrates that can't be broken down and absorbed by the small intestine. This fiber reaches the large intestine intact, without any energy being absorbed into the body. Fiber is therefore not classed as a carbohydrate on food nutritional labels.

There are two types of fibers: insoluble and soluble. Insoluble fiber does not dissolve in water. Our digestive system or bacteria can't use this fiber; instead, it acts as a sweep to help scrub and keep the gut clean. Insoluble fiber can be found in wholegrain products.

Soluble fiber, on the other hand, acts as nutrition for our good bacteria. It can be found in fruit, berries, vegetables, and oats. Water-soluble fiber is classified as a prebiotic.

#### A CRIME AGAINST OUR FIBER CONTRACT

Even if the concept of consuming prebiotics sounds new, foods rich in prebiotic fiber have been part of our diet since prehistoric times. It's not really that strange. When humans and other multicellular animals made our first contracts with bacteria to be hosted in the gut, the conditions of our contract were based on fiber—we were unable to digest fiber, but bacteria could, so the deal was done. So, it shouldn't come as a surprise that our bacteria now protest against the modern diet, which is lacking in fiber. It's us, not our unicellular friends, who have broken the contract. Researchers estimate that our prehistoric forebears ate as much as 135 grams of prebiotic fibers every day—that is twenty-two times as much as our daily recommended dose of a measly 6 grams of prebiotics. How did our original and natural intake of prebiotics reduce so drastically? A big problem, of course, is that the modern food industry has successfully removed a large part of fiber from our food (see p. 84). With our new knowledge on the importance of prebiotics to our gut health and brain, it is high time to incorporate bacteria-nourishing fiber back into our diet. Every prebiotic choice you make will strengthen your gut flora and probably brain—and as a bonus you might even improve your mood.

#### THE FANTASTIC BUTYRIC ACID—AGAIN

Prebiotic fiber is the favorite food of good bacteria, which in return produce healthy fatty acids and vitamins for their human hosts. Butyric acid is one such super acid that some bacteria produce as a healthy by-product. Apart from its anti-inflammatory properties, it has even been shown to reduce hunger hormones and suppress glucose and insulin (and, therefore, fat storage). Butyric acid also helps to build the gut's inner walls and repair gut leakage. Butyric acid affects the brain by stimulating the production of feel-good substances like serotonin. In addition, it reduces the pH levels in the gut, which inhibit the growth of harmful bacteria that would otherwise produce toxins like ammonia from our food. The list goes on. In summary: make sure you feed your good bacteria with plenty of fiber to get the fantastic anti-inflammatory butyric acid in return!

#### INULIN (PREBIOTIC)

Inulin is a big source of prebiotics that occurs naturally in many plants and vegetables. Inulin is sweet and gelatinous and shouldn't be confused with the blood-sugar-regulating hormone insulin. Inulin is often used as a replacement for sugar and fat within the food industry, so look carefully at the contents of nutritional labels next time. If inulin is listed, you can enjoy the sweetness with a good conscience in the knowledge that you are feeding your good bacteria.

Apart from strengthening you gut flora, inulin helps to reduce constipation, reduce the risk of heart disease by lowering blood lipids, and strengthen your skeleton. In one study, the uptake of calcium in girls increased by almost 20 percent after taking inulin. Researchers believe that inulin can prevent osteoporosis later in life, at least in women. Even if exotic vegetables like chicory, salsify, and yams are known for their high concentration of insulin, there are also more well-known and easily available vegetables with a lot of inulin. I have placed them into four groups:

**Onion:** yellow onion, red onion, garlic, scallions, leeks, chives
**Roots:** Jerusalem artichoke, globe artichoke, fennel, beetroot
**Leaves:** endives, dandelion leaves, arugula
**Other:** green bananas, asparagus, lentils, beans, broccoli

The amount of inulin in these vegetables varies. Green bananas contain only 1 percent of inulin, which means you need half a kilogram of green bananas to reach the daily recommended dose of 6 grams of inulin. It might be easier to get your daily dose as a supplement—browse your local health food store or pharmacy for inulin powder.

In addition, half the amount of inulin in vegetables gets lost through cooking, so account for more if you are cooking your food. Sample, experiment, and introduce these jewels of nature into your diet, and both your gut flora and brain will thank you. (If you are not used to it, you might have to introduce the inulin a little at a time).

#### RESISTANT STARCH (PREBIOTICS)

Resistant starch is another important group in prebiotics. As the name suggests, these foods withstand being digested and absorbed by the small intestine, therefore counting as fiber. Once in the large intestine, they act as food to our good bacteria, which produce the anti-inflammatory butyric acid from the starch. Apart from greatly enhancing gut flora, this super fiber reduces the risk of colon cancer in meat-eaters.

Potato, pasta, and bananas are typically not considered “diet” foods, but if you eat them in the right way, their resistant starch may even help you lose weight. Resistant starch passes through the gut without affecting blood sugar and insulin, making us feel full for longer, reducing hunger pangs, decreasing the uptake of calories, and increasing the burning of fat. So, how is resistant starch created? When pasta, rice, and potato cools down, the sugar chains and starch become resistant. For example, a medium-large cooked potato contains 19 grams of carbohydrates, but when it’s cooled, 4 grams of resistant starch is produced and the calories reduce from around 76 to 66. New studies also show that cold pasta, potato, and rice become even more resistant after being warmed up. So, don’t be afraid of carbohydrates; just make sure you prepare them correctly by cooling them and then warming them up again. In other words, it's the perfect opportunity for a packed lunch. Of course, I also had to include my favorite recipe for kimchi fried rice, made from kimchi and cold, leftover rice (see p. 154). Here is a list of foods with resistant starch, in a rough order of highest to lowest:

Potato flour
Green bananas
Cashew nuts
Uncooked oats
Peas (cooked)
Lentils (cooked)
Cold, cooked potato
Cold, cooked brown rice
Wholemeal bread

Potato flour contains the most resistant starch (72 percent), but it can be hard to consume, even if prebiotic devotees mix potato flour in cold water and drink it to optimize their gut flora! The potato flour must not be warmed up as it will then turn into normal starch. What is the recommended daily dose for resistant starch? Studies show that 15 to 30 grams (around 2 to 4 tablespoons of potato flour) is a suitable amount. Note that for people with a sensitive stomach or an overgrowth of bacteria in the gut, this can be too much.

Why not add some cold potatoes to your smoothie? This way, you'll sort out your daily dose of resistant starch in a meal.

#### OLIGOSACCHARIDES (PREBIOTIC)

Oligosaccharides are the last group of prebiotic fiber that serves the important function of feeding our bacteria. Fructooligosaccharides (FOS), galactooligosaccharides (GOS), and even inulin are all important types of oligosaccharides. In addition to feeding probiotic bacteria, oligosaccharides have been shown to have promising psychobiotic effects, especially when it comes to stress-related issues. It is thought that oligosaccharides reduce anxiety, strengthen mental ability, and reduce stress-related responses. Interestingly, oligosaccharides are produced by probiotic bacteria—in other words, bacteria both produce and eat oligosaccharides.

GOS are actually the first type of prebiotic we ingest, constituting almost 90 percent of all prebiotics in breast milk and showing how important GOS are for infants.

FOS consist of short fructose chains, and they appear naturally in fruit and vegetables like garlic, yellow onion, leeks, chicory, Jerusalem artichoke, asparagus, and banana. Most of these fruits and vegetables also have high levels of inulin. FOS can be bought as a supplement, and they have long been popular as a sweetener in the food industry. To keep your gut flora in shape, a daily dose of 4 to 6 grams is recommended. A strong therapeutic dose is around 10 to 20 grams, which is divided into three doses and taken with a meal. High doses (more than 15 grams) of FOS can cause gas, cramps, and diarrhea, which is why FOS intake should be gradually increased over a few weeks.

#### PREBIOTIC ADVICE

If you are not used to eating fiber, you should consider a few things. Try and get your fiber via food, as you will be guaranteed to get a variety of several types of prebiotics, which will feed many different bacterial species. A rich and diverse species is the best way to keep your gut flora and brain in top shape. In addition, you'll also get vitamins and strong antioxidants that have been shown to protect the gut flora against harmful bacteria. Generally, raw and unripe fruit and vegetables have more fiber than those that are cooked and ripe—for example, a green banana has a lot more fiber than a ripe banana. The best thing about prebiotic fiber is that harmful bacteria don't like it, which is why your good bacteria can eat it in peace and quiet, without worrying about an increase in competition. For each 100 grams of fiber you ingest, you produce 30 grams of beneficial bacteria—and remember that only 1 gram of fecal substance contains 100 billion bacteria. This means you can quickly increase good bacteria and push out bad bacteria by simply feeding your bacteria with plenty of prebiotic food.

Another benefit about getting prebiotics through food is that you reduce the risk of "overdosing"—you need to be careful with your prebiotic intake especially if you belong to the large population who has long survived on fiber-deficient white bread, pasta, and premade meals. It is enough for unaccustomed stomachs to get diarrhea and sulfur-smelling gas from 40 grams of inulin, which is not always appreciated by the people around you. The fact is that all types of fiber produce gas, so don't go too far and keep within the recommended dose. For example, the recommended daily intake for the prebiotic GOS is around 5 to 15 grams, and most people tolerate around 12 grams per day. If you still get swollen or gassy, take it easy and reduce the amount. If you suffer from more serious gut problems like IBS or IBD (inflammatory bowel disease), you need to be even more careful and possibly avoid fiber completely as often you need to heal your gut before introducing it again. Some people with IBS or IBD are forced to follow a special FODMAP diet during a certain period, which means ironically enough that you avoid food rich in probiotics and prebiotics. The good news is that a one-sided diet like this isn't meant for forever, and most people can return to a normal diet after healing their gut. Talk to a dietician or your doctor if you have any gut problems so you know what suits you.

### Eat more fermented foods (probiotics)

Most of the bacteria that have been confirmed by researchers to be effective can be found in fermented foods like yogurt and kimchi. Lactic acid bacteria, fermented bacteria, and probiotic bacteria are all the same thing, which makes sense—both fermenting and probiotics kill harmful bacteria. In the same way that harmful bacteria rots food if you don't ferment it correctly, the body also gets inflamed by bad bacteria if you don't take care of your gut flora. We have already paid a high price with our health due to our ignorance of the difference between good and bad bacteria, and hopefully our newfound fascination with our bacterial world hasn't come too late.

Over the years, every human culture has developed their own version of fermenting food, all of which feature good bacteria with a potential for psychobiotic effects. Stuffed with living bacteria that have been shown to boost the brain among other things, fermented food has also been shown to reduce social anxiety.

Pickling vegetables is a popular way to ferment food. A portion of sauerkraut or kimchi can contain up to a billion healthy bacteria or more. Unfortunately, most varieties found in stores are pasteurized (without living bacteria), so feel free to use my recipes for kimchi to get your intake of healthy bacteria (pages 140–154).

First and foremost, the process of fermenting is a lifesaver that has helped humans to conserve and protect food against mold and disease-carrying bacteria for over five thousand years. Nearly all food can be fermented—vegetables, fruit, milk, fish, and meat. Did you know that prosciutto and salami are both fermented meats?

Let's visit the cultures most famous for fermenting, starting with the East.

#### JAPAN AND KOREA—KOMBUCHA AND KIMCHI

Both Japanese and Korean kitchens contain fermented foods, such as soy, miso, tempeh, gochujang, and, last but not least, kombucha and kimchi. Kombucha and kimchi consistently top the list of probiotic foods, showing that they are considered to be some of the world's healthiest foods. I've shared some of my best recipes for kombucha and kimchi later on in the book, all to strengthen your brain (pp. 156–171)!

#### COFFEE, BEER, AND CHOCOLATE

Good news! Many of the best things in life are fermented, such as chocolate, cheese, yogurt, beer, wine, coffee, tea, and bread. Many of us can attest to the fact that a good cup of coffee and a piece of dark chocolate have a clearly positive effect on our mood!

Depending on what you feed your gut bacteria, fermentation can create wonders both for your health and taste buds. Soy and miso are made from beans, and so are coffee and chocolate, and if you feed yeast cells with sugar you produce alcohol, taking care of harmful bacteria along the way. If you then feed alcohol to bacteria, you produce vinegar, which in turn kills harmful bacteria. The same species of yeast has been used throughout the years to brew beer and proof bread, and even if these delicacies are not always healthy, from time immemorial we have brought fermented bacteria into our kitchens, restaurants, breweries, and bakeries.

#### FRANCE, PASTEUR, AND WINE

Even wine is produced by using the bacteria found naturally on grapes. In France, the country of wine lovers, Louis Pasteur discovered that the wrong type of bacteria could destroy wine, and he also found out which types of yeast, temperatures, and other conditions were needed to ferment grapes to wine. His work probably saved the French wine industry, which we are grateful for today. Pasteur then continued to research the effect of bacteria on food and humans. Among other things, he discovered that heating milk and other liquids killed bacteria. This process is used widely by the food industry today and has of course been named after Pasteur: pasteurization.

#### BULGARIA, METCHNIKOFF, AND YOGURT

Pasteur's Russian colleague Élie Metchnikoff is someone who had a great deal of enthusiasm when it came to investigating bacteria's positive effects on our health. He did this by studying the link between yogurt and aging. Metchnikoff was fascinated by Bulgarian farmers whose long lives, he suspected, depended on the fermented milk known as yogurt. These days, of course, we know that several types of lactic acid bacteria have psychobiotic effects. Metchnikoff subsequently won the Nobel prize for his pioneering work on the immune system and is said to have eaten yogurt for the rest of his life.

How is yogurt made? Yogurt, kefir, sour milk, and other types of fermented milk are produced by introducing bacteria from our two most common probiotic genera: *Lactobacillus bulgaricus* and *Streptococcus thermophilus*. In an optimal setting, the lactobacillus bacteria multiply and eat the lactose to produce lactic acid, which in turn ferments the milk and makes it sour. If, like me, you are lactose intolerant, you can still enjoy yogurt as most of the lactose is eaten up by the lactobacillus bacteria.



#### SUGAR-FREE AND FULL-FAT YOGURT

To create yogurt and sour milk, pasteurized milk is used, which means that all naturally occurring bacteria are eliminated through heat. After this process, living bacteria are added (*Lactobacillus bulgaricus* and *Streptococcus thermophilus*) to create yogurt. These days, many dairy producers add additional bacterial species to get stronger probiotic effects. It is therefore worth reading the list of ingredients to see which bacteria have been added. Extra points go to those who have added vitamin D, as research shows that vitamin D strengthens the probiotic effect in lactic acid bacteria in yogurt. Look at the label carefully to also make sure that bacteria have been added if the yogurt had been pasteurized. Look also for sugar content. Many types of yogurt are packed with sugar, which essentially removes its psychobiotic effects. Choose a brand without added sugar, but don't be afraid to choose a version with more fat. In a large study on 14,500 people, consumption of full-fat yogurt reduced the risk of depression, while non-fat yogurt did not reduce the risk. In summary, if you want to boost your brain with yogurt, choose natural, sugar-free yogurt with fat content! If you are vegan, allergic to milk, or lactose intolerant, you can find other variants on yogurt made from oat, soy, or coconut milk. In these cases, you should still choose natural, sugar-free, and full-fat yogurt varieties if you can. Since many of us already eat yogurt for breakfast, it's not so difficult to get living bacteria inside our guts on a daily basis.

#### PROBIOTIC ADVICE

If the health of your gut flora has improved due to diet, it's important to continue to feed it probiotic food. In other words, get into new food habits. Give it some time, a few attempts, and be kind to yourself and dare to experiment until you slowly but surely change the bacterial constitution of your gut flora. When you have made some progress, your good bacteria will be so vast in numbers that you'll start to crave fermented food—at least this is what researchers believe. What a positive spiral to get into!

#### PSYCHOBIOTIC GUIDANCE FROM THE PAST

How can we adapt the healthy diets of our forebears to our modern world? One easy way is to examine how our remaining hunter-gatherer tribes in Tanzania and the Amazon eat (see p. 83)—the food they consume reflects the dietary philosophy of our ancestors who hunted ten thousand years ago. The following guidelines summarize this food wisdom from the past.

#### EAT MAINLY PLANTS

Even if it is difficult for us to access a large variety of plants like the Yanomamis do, it is important to increase diversity as much as you can. If you can see all the colors of the rainbow on your plate and avoid dull, colorless food, you're doing well. Eating colorful plant-based food is also a surefire way to get enough fiber and other important nutrients, such as antioxidants, in your body. If you want to eat meat, treat it as a side or supplement, like people do in Japan or Korea, rather than as a main ingredient.

#### EAT THE WHOLE FRUIT AND VEGETABLE

Eat the whole fruit rather than drinking it as juice. This way, you'll retain important fiber that has been shown to stimulate the production of anti-inflammatory butyric acid. Similarly, eat the whole vegetable rather than just parts of it. For example, many people eat just the florets of broccoli or cauliflower, missing out on the fiber from their leaves and stalk. Additionally, pick fruits and vegetables that have not been sprayed with chemicals as research shows that the pesticides and antibiotics in fertilizer damage our gut flora.



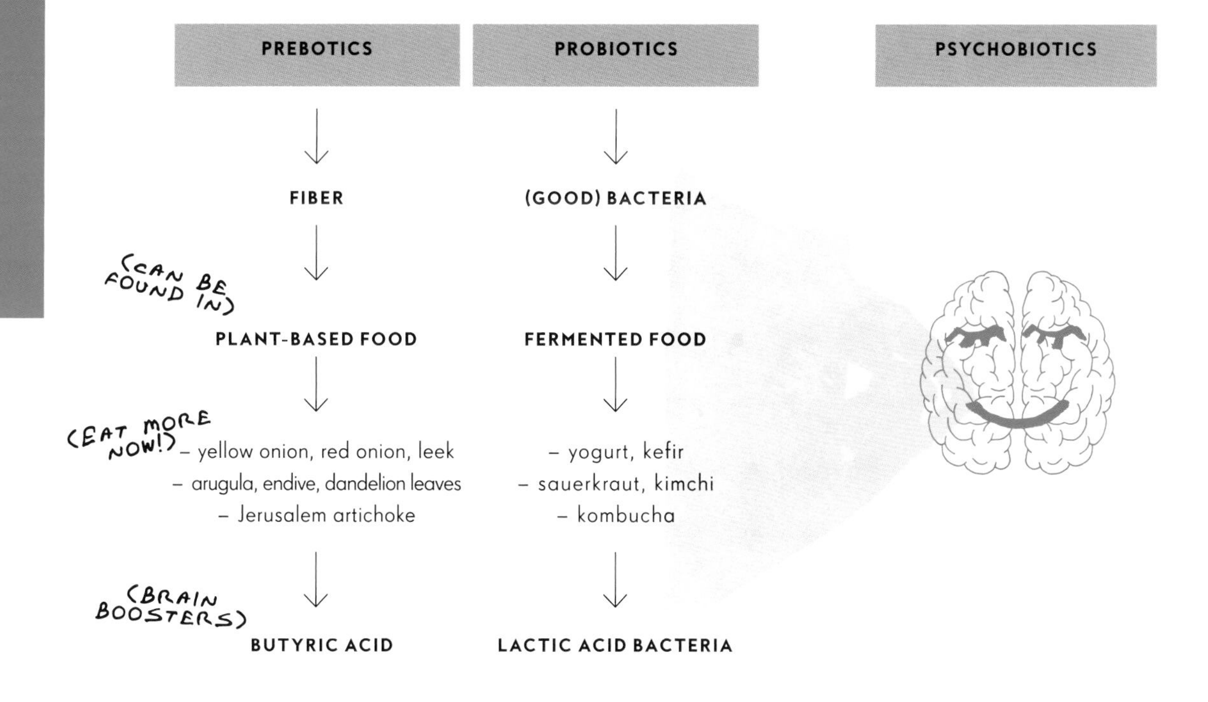

#### EAT UNPROCESSED FOOD

Eat as many natural foods as possible, which refers to food that has not been sprayed with chemicals or overprocessed, e.g., premade meals. Also reduce foods that are based on grain and flour (cookies, bread, and pasta), which barely existed before the agricultural revolution. Natural foods mean eating lots of raw vegetables and fruits so you can get plenty of prebiotic fiber and other healthy substances like antioxidants, vitamins, and minerals. Eating natural, whole foods instead of overprocessed foods from the food industry is a new trend that is, thankfully, growing on a global scale.

#### DIVERSITY, DIVERESITY, DIVERSITY

Studies show that it doesn't really matter what exact bacteria colonize our gut. Our gut's constitution depends on our context—where we live, what we eat, and so on—and varies from person to person. What we can be sure of is that gut flora is reflected in the food we eat, which varies enormously around the world. If there is one message that researchers are pushing, it's: diversity, diversity, diversity. This means the more types of food you eat, the more bacteria will enrich your gut; while the fewer types of food you eat, the fewer bacterial species will live in your gut, which contributes to an unbalanced gut flora and major disturbances in the dialogue between the gut and brain. This is why colorless, bland post-workout foods (like rice and chicken or tuna) or one-sided diets that eliminate foods (like many of the trendy diets these days) are not recommended if you want to boost your brain, Instead, consume well-balanced meals with lots of vegetables and fruit in all the colors of the rainbow. If you are an omnivore, complement your meal with lean meat or, even better, with fish (preferably wild). It's really about common sense and just like your mother or grandmother said: eat more vegetables and less cookies and ice cream.

#### POPPING PSYCHOBIOTIC PILLS

Probiotics are defined as a living microorganism that in large enough amounts provide positive health effects to their human host. When this includes positive health effects that boost the brain, probiotics are called *psychobiotics*. When you mention the word *probiotics*, there's a big chance that many people think about good bacteria that comes in the form of a pill. And when people wish to fix something like an unhealthy gut flora, their first tendency might be to simply pop a pill. But the situation is not as easy as just "fixing your gut flora" with a pill, as not all probiotic products have been shown to be effective.

Researchers are united in the fact that the best and safest way to get living bacteria inside you is via the food you eat. If you still choose to pop a probiotic pill, make sure to read the label carefully and follow the rules below.

#### WATCH OUT FOR FAKES

Commercial players have not been slow in jumping on the gut flora bandwagon, which has hit us over the past few years. The market has literally exploded with probiotic products, and not all of them can be trusted. A sobering study showed that out of the market's thirteen most common probiotics, only four contained what the labels said they contained. Several studies have also found considerably lower numbers of bacteria in probiotic products while others did

**Soki Choi reflects over diet trends and the letter F**

For a long time, trendy diets, which come and go like fashion, have bothered me. Eating your way to a healthier and stronger brain is about first trying to repair the damage that the four revolutions have caused our gut flora. Therefore, there is no quick fix; instead the solution is a lifestyle change that takes time. In a world of information overload, I've come up with a mnemonic to help you remember the best way to eat your way to a healthy lifestyle: think of the letter F as in Fiber, Fermented Food, Fish, Fasting, and color-Ful, and you'll get there!



not contain the bacterial species they claimed to on their labels—including potentially harmful bacteria. It is worth checking that you are buying a trusted product, especially since they are not cheap.

#### KEEP THEM CHILLED IN THE FRIDGE

Living bacteria die as soon as they get too warm, which is why probiotics can get damaged on the way to the store or your home. Living bacteria need to be delivered in an unbroken chilled chain. A broken chilled chain, which can easily happen, means you risk buying an expensive jar of ineffective bacteria. Therefore, it's important that you store them in the fridge unless they are freeze-dried supplements, in which case they'll survive.

#### IT'S IMPOSSIBLE TO OVERDOSE

In order for the probiotics to have an effect, you need to get enough of it—meaning, several billion living bacteria. In order to be counted as living, each bacterium needs to be able to divide into two so they can form a new colony. The typical unit for probiotics is known as CFU or *colony forming unit*. The sad reality is that less than a third will survive the torturous journey through your gut, where corrosive stomach acid can easily kill them. This is why it is normal for each capsule to contain tens of billions of CFUs. Compared to medication, for which there is an exact dose, no exact doses have been established for probiotics. In other words, in contrast to medicine, it is almost impossible to overdose on probiotic bacteria, especially if taken via food.

#### CHOOSE A CAPSULE

Capsules are better than tablets as capsules have been shown to be more resistant to the stomach's digestive juices—unless they are freeze-dried tablets. Most probiotics come in capsules.

Prebiotics, on the other hand, are normally sold in powder form since you need larger amounts of fiber compared to probiotics. Prebiotic fiber is easy to stir into yogurt, smoothies, or juices. Fiber also doesn't need the same rigorous cold storage process as probiotic bacteria. Although prebiotic fiber is not "alive," prebiotics are still classified as psychobiotics as they feed living beneficial bacteria (see p. 90).

#### A COMPLEMENT TO FOOD

Researchers agree on the fact that the best and safest way to get plenty of living bacteria inside you is through food. When consuming probiotics through food, It is important not to heat the food too much as that kills the bacteria. Even if you choose to stick to the pill bottle for your probiotics, you still need to feed your gut flora prebiotic fiber that is easiest to get through food (vegetable, fruit, legumes, etc.). Your brain-boosting bacteria need to multiply to be effective and keep harmful bacteria at bay, so make sure that your probiotics supplements are just that—a supplement to a fiber-rich diet.



## *The future of medicine*

In the not too distant future, many experts believe we will have capsules with customized psychobiotic bacteria meant to treat autism, ADHD, anxiety, depression, and maybe even Alzheimer's and Parkinson's. For the first time, this completely new medical paradigm is challenging pharmacological therapy, which has dominated the treatment of psychiatric disorders since the 1950s. Even if there is a long way to go, preliminary research shows that bacteria could have the capacity to treat psychiatric problems in the future. The hope is that psychoactive bacteria will demonstrate that they have the capacity to be used like Prozac and Valium, but with fewer side effects. To find the right dosage and combination will prove tricky, as there are thousands of bacterial species to choose from that have to interact with your existing gut flora. Even small differences in lifestyle can mean that you'll have a completely different set of psychobiotic needs than another person. There is a lot left to do, but it's very exciting that research into psychobiotics is challenging the current medical status quo. And because I'm an impatient person, I will now invite you into the future of medicine in this chapter, where we will visit the colorful Santa's workshop of scientists, doctors, and companies from all over the world who are currently testing and experimenting with medication of the future.

**FECAL TRANSPLANT (STOOL TRANSFER)**

Food and supplements are the normal way to get living bacteria inside your body, but there is another more invasive method—a stool transfer, which in medicinal terms is called a *fecal transplant*. However disgusting it sounds, the transfer of fresh feces from a healthy person to a patient seems to be the most successful way to treat serious infections like *Clostridium difficile* (*C. diff*). The huge progress with *C. diff* infections has meant that doctors are now testing fecal transplants for IBS, Crohn's disease, leaky gut syndrome, and even diabetes and obesity. Stools from healthy donors have been shown to help improve the insulin sensitivity of people with diabetes. In addition, the stool transfer from an "extroverted and exploring" mouse to an "introverted and shy" mouse resulted in the "introvert" mouse gaining the same "extroverted" behaviors as their donor. The whole idea that stool transfers can change behavior has absolutely floored researchers and doctors. Let's take a closer look at fecal transplants within three exciting contexts: *C. diff*, mental illness, and autism.

**FECAL TRANSLPLANTS AND *C-DIFF***

*C. diff* (*Clostridium difficile*) is a type of gut bacteria that affects half a million Americans in a year and over seven thousand Swedes each year. *C. diff* infections result in bloody diarrhea, high fever, stomach cramps, and nausea, which can continue for several years. The death rate is 20 percent in serious cases, and many times it is necessary to remove parts of the gut and have a colostomy bag for life. In 2015, *C. diff* killed approximately twenty-nine thousand Americans within thirty days of the diagnosis, and it has also taken the lives of more Swedes than the infamous multiresistant bacteria MRSA. A *C. diff* infection is dangerous even when you take antibiotics. The antibiotics will kill good bacteria while the *C. diff* survives, since it is extremely resistant to antibiotics, which is why it is often called "the last bug standing." The bacteria create spores, allowing it to survive for a long time and get stuck in health care environments for years, making it extremely contagious.

Luckily, even though a fecal transplant is a relatively new tool, it has been shown to be miraculously successful against *C. diff* infections. In a study, 94 percent of all patients got completely better after a stool transfer. A fecal transplant is therefore an established and effective treatment against *C. diff*.

**FECAL TRANSPLANTS AND MENTAL ILLNESS**

Fecal transplants have been shown to transfer symptoms of depression and anxiety between animals. The amazing thing is that the transfer can also occur between animals and humans, which goes to show that some bacteria are universal. For example, healthy mice displayed anxious behavior after having received feces from an anxious person. Leading researchers from University College Cork in Ireland reported that a depressed patient had gotten rid of their depressive symptoms only a few hours after receiving a fecal transplant. Even if larger studies are needed for more conclusive evidence, researchers believe that fecal transplants will soon be able to treat depression and anxiety. Even now, we can confirm that bacteria definitely have the ability to affect our mood. If you should ever need a fecal transplant, it is wise to also do a psychological screening of your donor so your gut flora doesn't accidentally take over "melancholic" bacteria from a donor who suffers from depressive symptoms. The fact that fecal transplants can affect our behavior, brain, and mental health has shocked the world of research, opening the doors to something that many believe will be a new paradigm in medicine.

#### FECAL TRANSPLANTS AND AUTISM

Apart from stress-related illnesses like depression and anxiety, fecal transplants have also been tested on neuropsychiatric diagnoses, such as autism.

A noted study spread like wildfire through the world of autism after a fecal transplant drastically reduced autism-like behavior in mice. When the stools from mice with autism-like behavior were transferred into "normal" mice, the normal mice began to behave like their "autistic" donors. What was even more bizarre was that this autism-like behavior disappeared when beneficial bacteria were reintroduced into the mice from a healthy human. Researchers believe this shows that substances that produce bacteria (in stools) can reach the brain and change behaviors in both normal and abnormal mice. This study was considered well-designed and given a lot of attention from researchers, as well as parents of children with autism and companies on standby to develop groundbreaking therapies for autism. The enthusiasm grew when a smaller study on children with autism showed that fecal transplants led to an 80 percent improvement of both gut problems and certain behaviors related to autism (see from p. 69).

Even if fecal transplants are still classed as experimental, many are hopeful that patients with autism will be treated with fecal transplants in the near future. Even if "only" a small group of patients have improved symptoms, it would still mean a scientific breakthrough.

#### DON'T DIY IN THE KITCHEN!

Today there are many do-it-yourself tips on YouTube for those brave people who want to try fecal transplants themselves! However tempting it is, it is not a good idea to try a stool transfer at home. Remember that gut flora is considered an organ in its own right—you would never transplant an organ in the kitchen, would you? One of the big problems is that there are so many bacterial species in feces, which makes it hard to know which are good and which are poisonous and dangerous (even in a laboratory environment). For people who are seriously ill, a fecal transplant can be an alternative medical treatment that should be done within a hospital setting. In other words, don't conduct a DIY fecal transplant!

### Microbirthing

Children born by cesarean section have been shown to be at a higher risk of suffering from allergies, asthma, and even autism. Many women who give birth via cesarean section have jumped on the bandwagon of a trend known as *vaginal seeding* or *microbirthing*, which is when a cotton swab is dipped in vaginal fluid and rubbed over the baby's face, eyes, and mouth immediately after the C-section. The idea is to cover the child with the bacteria that would have covered their bodies if they had been born vaginally, and mothers hope this will kick-start their babies' immune systems in order to reduce the risk of allergies, asthma, and autism. Skeptical researchers suggest that there is no evidence of long-term benefits and that it can cause dangerous infections. They feel that more studies in "safe, controlled clinical environments" are needed before microbirthing can be recommended. As with everything else in life, the issue is about weighing the risks against potential benefits, and most people agree that C-sections give children a worse gut flora compared to vaginal births.

## Customized food

Medication and trendy diets are all based on the idea that we all react in the same way to food, but as I've previously stated, everyone is different. We will react differently to the same food, even if our genes and the environment are, as far as we can see, the same. Researchers believe it is just a matter of time before customized probiotics based on the mapping of gut bacteria will become available to everyone. Already several companies have invested in systems that provide information on tailormade diets with the aim of optimizing an individual's health—masses of unique personal data is placed into an algorithm, which then spits out customized dietary recommendations. The data can come from different tests (stool, urine, blood, etc.), measurements (blood sugar, blood pressure, sleep, etc.) and other relevant information (age, sex, weight, height, heredity information, etc.). You would need to write down exactly what you eat and when you eat, as well as your exercise routine and other activities over a period of time. This method requires a big investment on the individual's behalf and so will probably be of less interest to people who are seriously ill, where dietary changes are not a guaranteed form of treatment, but of more interest to those who are slightly ill and suffering from Western illnesses like metabolic syndrome. Metabolic syndrome includes being overweight and having high blood sugar, high blood pressure, and elevated blood lipids, which can easily lead to type 2 diabetes and cardiovascular disease. It is a broad "pre-disease" condition that every fourth person over the age of thirty suffers from. About 34 percent of American adults are believed to suffer from metabolic syndrome. Did you know that heart disease is the leading cause of death for both men and women in America, causing about one in four deaths (610,000 deaths) every year? Meanwhile, in Sweden, as many as four out of ten people die of cardiovascular disease. Together with mental health problems, metabolic syndrome is a growing epidemic that the health care of today is not equipped to treat. Instead, our focus is on treating people who have already gotten sick. The good news is that you can personally take steps to prevent metabolic syndrome and even mental illness by changing your diet and other lifestyle habits—by focusing on the constitution of your gut flora. Modern science has finally caught up with what Hippocrates understood 2,500 years ago: food is medicine.

### YOGURT BY PRESCRIPTION

In the United States, it is common for doctors to "prescribe" yogurt in combination with antibiotics. This is to compensate for the unavoidable elimination of good bacteria that antibiotics and even other medicine cause. It shouldn't take too long until it also becomes common practice in other countries such as Sweden.

It's mainly *Lactobacillus casei* (*L. casei*), which is found in yogurt, that helps to replenish good bacteria. *L. casei* also has the capacity to increase the amount of Bifidobacteria, which further strengthens the probiotic effect. Even *L. paracasei*, which is found in yogurt and probiotic cocktails, has been shown to reduce pain levels and stress in our gut caused by antibiotics. Simply put, it is smart to eat yogurt, kimchi, and kombucha to replenish your good bacteria whenever you take antibiotics or other medication.

#### BACTERIA AS OUR NEW MINI-DOCTORS

It is believed that future medicine will become more and more customized ("personalized medicine"), meaning that medication, including food, is developed and adapted for each individual's unique needs. Researchers are also trying to produce more accurate bacteria to target specific ailments by redesigning the bacteria's genes. This is done by cutting and pasting the genome sequence back and forth in bacteria. The hope is to produce bacteria that work like mini-doctors that, when they reach our gut, can produce substances that treat, or even cure, diseases such as diabetes, obesity, depression, and anxiety. In this case, genetically redesigned bacteria would be ingested in the form of "programmed yogurt." Since this involves tinkering with genes, there are ethical implications with this process, meaning it might take some time before the general public will accept these new treatments. Regardless, it is very exciting and much of the research is already underway!

## *Your bacterial guide to a stronger brain*

Several important projects are being conducted all over the world on which bacteria can enhance the brain and/or reduce mental health problems, i.e., psychobiotics. Psychobiotic bacteria generally come from two genera: *Bifidobacterium* and *Lactobacillus*. It is common for researchers and producers to combine species from both these genera into one psychobiotic cocktail. Even if larger studies are needed to continue this research, early studies on both animals and humans suggest that "normal" lactic acid bacteria are effective against mental health disorders. To navigate around this exciting new world, I've included a list of the most researched psychobiotic bacteria. Refer to this for your own information to guide you to a healthier gut flora and a stronger brain.

#### 1. *BIFIDOBACTERIUM ANIMALIS LACTIS*

*B. animalis lactis* has been shown to improve moods when taken in combination with *L. bulgaricus*, *L. lactis*, and *S. thermophiles*. The closely related *B. animalis* is good for people suffering from constipation, diarrhea, ulcerative colitis, IBS, and other stress-related gut problems. *B. animalis* also acts as a nutrient for other beneficial bifidobacteria and lactobacteria, increasing the psychobiotic effect.

#### 2. *BIFIDOBACTERIUM BIFIDUM*

If you were born vaginally, you are guaranteed to have received *B. bifidum* from your mother. It is one of the first bacteria that is introduced into a newborn's body when they move through the birth canal. *B. bifidum* helps prevent diarrhea and knocks out dangerous bacteria such as *E. coli* and the yeast candida. Interestingly, ingesting *B. bifidum* together with *L. acidophilus* and *L. casei* over a period of eight weeks has been shown to help people with severe depression.

#### 3. *BIFIDOBACTERIUM BREVE*

*B. breve* displays big similarities with *B. longum*, but there are a few interesting differences: *B. breve* has a stronger effect on anxiety, and *B. longum* has more antidepressant effects. Both bacterial species have been shown to be as effective against anxiety and depression as the antidepressant escitalopram (also known as Cipralex or Lexapro) in studies on animals. If lactic acid bacteria could compete successfully with antidepressants, it would be a revolutionary development.

#### 4. *BIFIDOBACTERIUM LONGUM (INFANTIS)*

*B. longum* reduces stress via the vagus nerve and the neuroendocrine system. *B. longum* can even reduce depression thanks to its beneficial effect on the hippocampus. *B. longum* also increases your memory, your cognitive capacity, and even your ability to handle stress under pressure, which is why it is of interest to healthy people who just want to enhance their productiveness. *B. longum* can be found naturally in yogurt and kefir.

#### 5. *LACTOBACILLUS ACIDOPHILUS*

*L. acidophilus* reduces intense anxiety by knocking out anxiety-enhancing bacteria. It can even prevent diarrhea, bacterial overgrowth (SIBO), and inflammation. In addition, it has painkilling effects. *L. acidophilus* is probably the most popular and common bacteria in probiotic products. You can find it in fermented food such as yogurt and sauerkraut.

#### 6. *LACTOBACILLUS CASEI*

A noted study showed that people with depression showed clear improvements after only ten days of eating yogurt containing *L. casei*. Even patients suffering from chronic fatigue experienced less anxiety and better gut health after taking *L. casei*. *L. casei* has also been shown to be very useful to treat diarrhea caused by antibiotics and *C. diff* infections. In addition, *L. casei* has an ability to increase the amount of bifidobacteria, which not only strengthens the psychobiotic effect but also demonstrates that a diverse mix of good bacteria can work well together. *L. casei* can be found in fermented milk products like different types of cheese and yogurt.

#### 7. *LACTOBACILLUS DELBRUECKII* SUBSP. *BULGARICUS*

This type of lactic acid bacteria is mainly known for reducing inflammation and strengthening the signals of our happy molecule serotonin. In addition, the bacteria has been shown to reduce blood pressure, fortify the immune system, and improve mood. It has also been shown to reduce anxiety. It can be found in fermented products like kimchi and yogurt.

#### 8. *LACTOBACILLUS PLANTARUM*

*L. plantarum* is a popular bacteria among probiotic producers. This type of lactic acid bacteria has been shown to reduce gut pain in patients with IBS and reduce inflammation and soy allergies. Apart from knocking out dangerous species like clostridia and enterococcus, *L. plantarum* also helps to boost the level of good bifidobacteria. In studies on animals, it has also been shown to increase memory and ever reduce age-related memory loss. *L. plantarum* can easily be found in fermented vegetables, such as sauerkraut and kimchi.

#### 9. *LACTOBACILLUS REUTERI*

*L. reuteri* is an interesting bacterial species with several unexpected psychobiotic properties. *L. reuteri* has, among other things, corrected autism-like socialization problems in newborn mice whose mothers had been fed an extremely high-fat diet. *L. reuteri* has been shown to increase the levels of oxytocin (bonding hormone) in both mice and humans. This psychobiotic bacteria also acts like an antibiotic as it is effective in killing harmful bacteria, with the ability to also quickly colonize the gut, which is good news. In addition, it can help to prevent heart disease by lowering bad cholesterol (LDL), reducing pain and associated anxiety, increasing the hormone that suppresses appetite, and reducing the hunger hormone, therefore helping you to reduce your calorie intake and lose weight. *L. reuteri* can be found in breast milk and fermented foods.

#### 10. *LACTOBACILLUS RHAMNOSUS*

Regular use of *L. rhamnosus* has been shown to reduce stress hormones, anxiety, nd depression, and even compulsions in studies on animals. Researchers believe this is because *L. rhamnosus* increases the neurotransmitter GABA, which is involved in problems related to anxiety and depression. This psychobiotic has been shown to be effective against IBS, which is highly comorbid with anxiety and depression. *L. rhamnosus* also produces many short-chain fatty acids, such as the anti-inflammatory butyric acid. Apart from healing the gut, butyric acid can penetrate the blood-brain barrier, providing an antidepressant effect right at the site of the brain. When combined with *L. paracasei*, it has been shown to minimize oxidative stress that occurs after high-intensity exercise. *L. rhamnosus* can be found in kimchi, yogurt, kefir, and even in Parmesan cheese.

## *Additional advice on psychobiotics*

Apart from the overall advice to eat plenty of food that is rich in fiber, as well as fermented and colorful foods, I want to finish off by giving you additional research-based advice on how to strengthen your brain through a healthier gut flora. My advice is not a one-stop "quick fix," but rather lifestyle tips. The idea behind improving the health of your gut flora is not just to fix the symptoms of a disease but instead to try to reach the cause behind it—an unbalanced gut flora.

#### MINIMIZE SUGAR INTAKE

By this point, I don't need to go into detail on what sugar does to our health. It comes as no surprise that sugar-loving bacteria cause disease. Fructose, which can be found in regular sugar and in plenty of the processed food we eat, increases bacterial toxins that can lead to liver damage, which compounds the problem when the liver is desperately trying to detoxify the body. Reduce sugar at all costs, and I promise you that your gut flora and brain will thank you.

#### MINIMIZE MEAT CONSUMPTION

Meat doesn't contain any probiotics or prebiotic fiber. Saturated fats, which can be found in meat and dairy products, have been shown to be inflammatory, causing stress to the gut. In addition, diets that feature a high consumption of meat and saturated fats (such as LCHF and Atkins) have been shown to change your gut flora for the worse. Interesting research has shown that mice that ate some meat—where the meat was of good quality with a lower fat content—showed signs of a higher diversity of bacterial species in their gut flora, reduced anxiety, and increased cognition than the mice that didn't eat any meat at all. This is probably because a greater variety of food leads to a larger variety of bacterial species, which is the signature of a healthy gut flora. In other words, it's worth mixing up different foods in your diet. That being said, most people in the West eat way too much red meat than what is recommended.

Personally, I avoid meat for ethical and environmental reasons. If you still want to eat meat to optimize your gut flora and brain health, a rule of thumb can be to do what they do in Asia—eat 80 percent of food from the plant kingdom and 20 percent from the animal kingdom, and remember that the meat should be of a really good quality with low fat content, and preferably wild or grass-fed.

#### MAKE SURE YOU GET SOME OMEGA-3

It's even better if your diet of meat consists of mostly fish. The polyunsaturated fat omega-3 is the complete opposite of saturated fat in meat. Apart from reducing inflammation, omega-3 has been shown to reduce the stress hormone cortisol and repair stress-related damage to the gut flora. In addition, omega-3 is essential to creating new nerves and synapses in the brain, which can enhance your cognitive and memory ability.

An easy way to recognize unhealthy saturated fats is that they are solids in room temperature (think about butter and the white fat in meat), while healthy polyunsaturated fats are runny oils that are liquid at room temperature. You can find omega-3 naturally in fish but also in olives, nuts, soybeans, and some oils. For example, when you consume olive oil, 80 percent of its fatty acids come into contact with your bacteria, which in turn produce healthy short-chain fatty acids that have an anti-inflammatory effect.

Fish is generally celebrated thanks to its high omega-3 content. Sadly, many fish contain toxic pollutants, such as quicksilver and dioxin. This is especially relevant to larger fish that live longer. As a result, it is better to eat fish like salmon, cod, and sardines. It is also worth noting that a strong gut flora can actually help to detoxify your body from mercury, while the opposite is true—a weak gut flora helps the body to concentrate mercury, especially in your brain. All the more reason to keep your gut flora in tip-top shape!

#### DON'T BE AFRAID OF CARBOHYDRATES

Fruits such as bananas, apples, and oranges have been shown to strengthen several beneficial bacteria. In other words, it is not a good idea to eliminate all carbohydrates, like some extreme diets such as LCHF and Atkins recommend—at least not if you want to optimize your gut flora, brain, and mental health. The fact is that complex carbohydrates in the form of cold potatoes and cold rice, as well as oligosaccharides and inulin, constitute prebiotic fiber that feeds your good bacteria and strengthen your brain. In addition, research shows that a well-composed gut flora can help you maintain a healthy weight—so don't be afraid of some carbohydrates!

#### FAST INTELLIGENTLY

If you want to eat to achieve a long life, calorie restrictions and fasting have been shown to help both animals and humans live longer. The practice of fasting seems to tell your cells to buck up. However strange it might sound, it kick-starts a process where your sick cells commit suicide to then be absorbed by your body. In medical terms, the process is called *autophagy* which means "to eat yourself." It was with this cannibalistic discovery that Japanese biologist Yoshinori Ohsumi was awarded the 2016 Nobel prize. Fasting reduces oxidative damage and inflammation, both of which are considered to contribute to aging.

The fact that evolution has made it beneficial to fast can also be seen in our guts. Fasting or greatly reducing your calorie intake has been shown to increase the level of the good bacteria akkermansia, which, among other things, reduces inflammation.

The good news is that you don't have to be especially strict, such as following a 5:2 diet or half-starving yourself. There is an easier and better way to fast: simply wait for twelve hours after dinner before you eat again the next day. If, for example, you eat at 7 p.m. in the evening, you can then eat breakfast at 7 a.m. at the earliest in the morning. Easy-peasy. This just means keeping away from the habit of snacking throughout the evening and in the night. If you can't do this long-term, even a shorter one-off fast has been shown to kick-start your gut flora, but the levels of good bacteria will reduce after about a week. It is best to try and get into a habit of a natural fast in your daily routine so you don't even need to think about it. Personally, the best time for me to fast is between dinner and breakfast. Try it and see if it suits you.

#### EXERCISE + FOOD = 1+1=3

It's not news that exercise is good for our health. Experts are united in the fact that regular exercise is good for the heart and muscles and increases life span. Scientists now also believe that exercise can have a direct effect on our brain depending on the constitution of our gut flora. New and exciting research shows that exercise can increase brain capacity in older people and improve depression by enhancing gut flora.

Exercise stimulates our bacteria's production of butyric acid. In light of a rapidly aging population all over the world, watching our levels of butyric acid, which can help sharpen memory, should be a focus for all of us.

When you exercise, you improve the health of your gut flora and subsequently your mental health. The amazing thing is that this also seems to go the other way—if your gut flora gets better through diet, your capacity for exercise can increase, allowing you to, say, run faster and longer. The fact that certain gut bacteria have shown to make mice run faster or swim for longer has attracted keen interest from the world of professional sports. Many sportspeople even get their gut flora profiled and update their diets, and taking kombucha or other probiotic drinks after exercise has become popular in the United States. We already know that food is the most decisive factor for our bacterial diversity, and even if it is too soon to discuss the exact link, exercise, too, seems to help fortify our gut flora.

Preliminary research doesn't only show that exercise can reduce anxiety and depression; it also shows that fiber-rich and fermented foods can do the same. Exercise and food are both cheap and freely available, so what's stopping you? Exercise regularly and eat a lot of psychobiotic food, and you will likely strengthen your brain twice over.

#### REDUCE STRESS

As we have seen, stress is devastating to our gut flora. Treating stress has become a huge industry, with countless self-help books and miracle homemade concoctions that claim to reduce stress levels, most of which have no proven effect. Luckily, research shows that the practice of meditation is effective in reducing stress, anxiety, and depression. And it's enough to meditate for 20 minutes for three days to feel an effect.

#### FOLLOW THIS ADVICE AT YOUR OWN PACE

Remember that gut flora is a living and dynamic ecosystem that is constantly changing through food, exercise, stress, and other lifestyle factors. Look at this advice like a smorgasbord where you can test one tip at a time or try whatever works for you. It is important to note that these tips are for generally healthy people (without a medical diagnosis) who have not yet become sick but who want to strengthen their brains and prevent mental illness. You must absolutely not stop taking any medication, therapy, or other treatments if you have a diagnosis. In many cases, medications are vital and save lives. Follow the prescriptions from your doctor, but supplement them with psychobiotic food. While waiting for more and larger studies to be conducted on humans, you can view these preventative tips as a health investment in your brain without nasty side effects.

Research shows that it takes around two months for a new habit to stick, so give yourself a pat on the back if you have managed to follow a piece of advice for two months. Then, move on to the next tip. My experience is that it is not really a viable strategy to try and do everything at once, even if you are raring to go. Don't forget that it is never too late to renew your gut flora. Each meal gives you a new chance to change your flora composition, which in time will reward you with better moods and a stronger brain. Good luck!

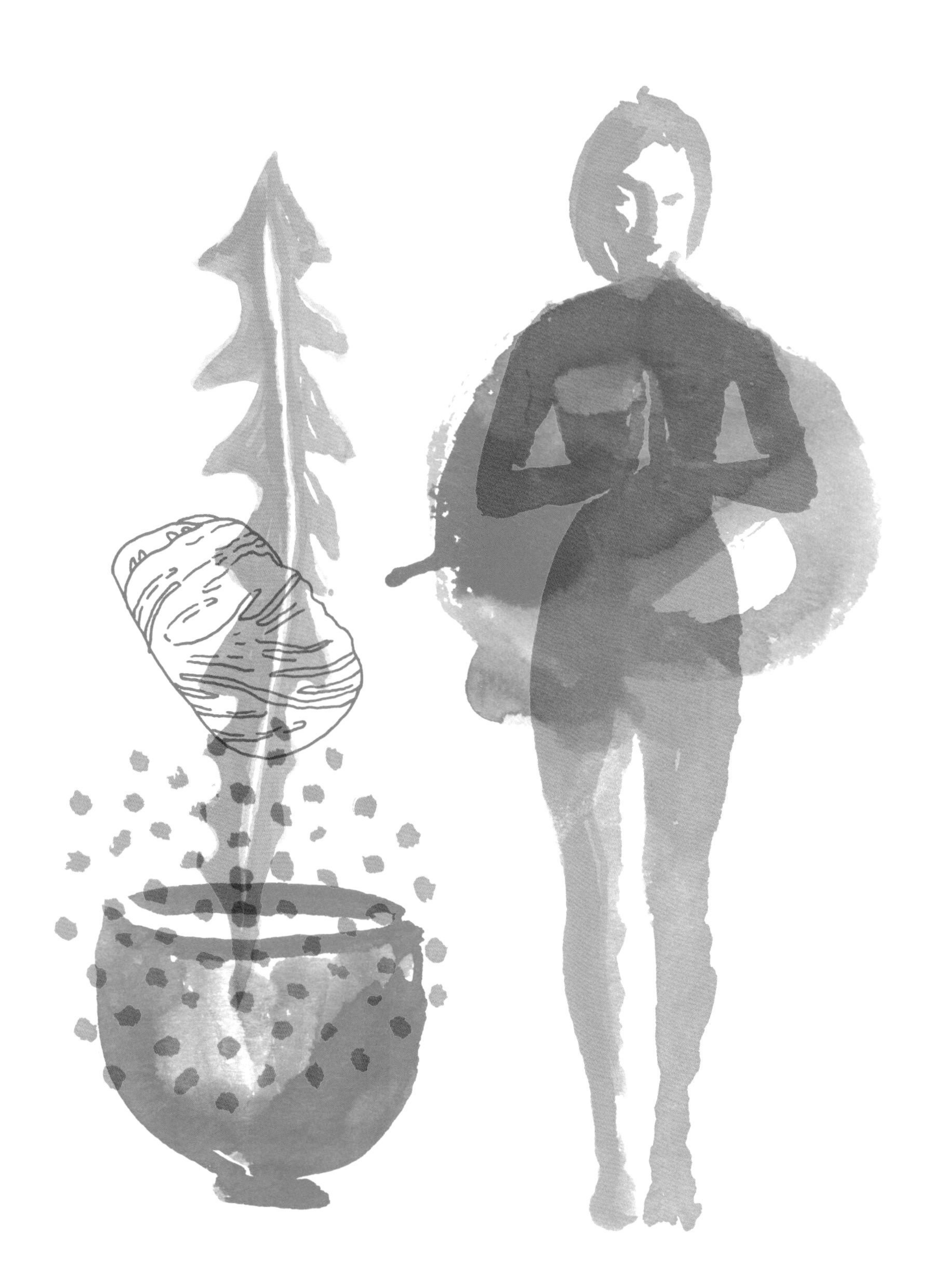

# *A summary of chapter 4*

**Ten psychobiotic tips to strengthen your brain**

1. Diversity, diversity, diversity: be inspired by our forebears who ate hundreds of different species—mostly from the plant kingdom. The more colorful vegetables and fruits you eat, the more bacterial species will enrich your gut, which is a sign of a strong gut-brain axis.

2. Eat lots of fiber: prebiotic fiber feeds your health-promoting bacteria, which create beneficial substances like the anti-inflammatory butyric acid.

3. Eat fermented foods: living lactic acid bacteria can be ingested via fermented foods that you can find in Mediterranean, Japanese, or Korean kitchens. In one gram of kimchi, you can find up to one hundred billion lactic acid bacteria.

4. Be careful with antibiotics: if you have to take antibiotics, replenish your gut with probiotic bacteria from fermented foods such as yogurt and kimchi.

5. Minimize your sugar intake: reduce soda, juice, sweets, and all other forms of sugar. Sugar feeds bad bacteria and bacterial toxins in the gut.

6. Eat less meat: animal saturated fats found in meat and dairy products have been shown to introduce stress to the gut and cause inflammation. Eat meat in moderation. On the other hand, polyunsaturated fats (omega-3) increase good bacteria, so eat fish, nuts, and plant-based oils.

7. Eat natural foods: chemical additives worsen both the thickness of the mucous membrane in your gut (leaky gut) and the diversity of species in your gut flora. Choose organic and unprocessed food without additives as much as you can.

8. Practice semi-fasting: fasting stimulates the growth of good bacteria. An easy way to get into a regular fasting routing is to make sure you go at least twelve hours without food between breakfast and dinner. Try and avoid snacking after dinner.

9. Exercise regularly: exercise has been shown to have a positive effect on your gut flora, which in turn can increase your training capacity.

10. Reduce stress: stress feeds harmful bacteria and promotes inflammation, which in turn can propagate in the brain and cause depression. Try meditating to reduce the harmful effects of stress.

CHAPTER 5

# Kimchi and kombucha

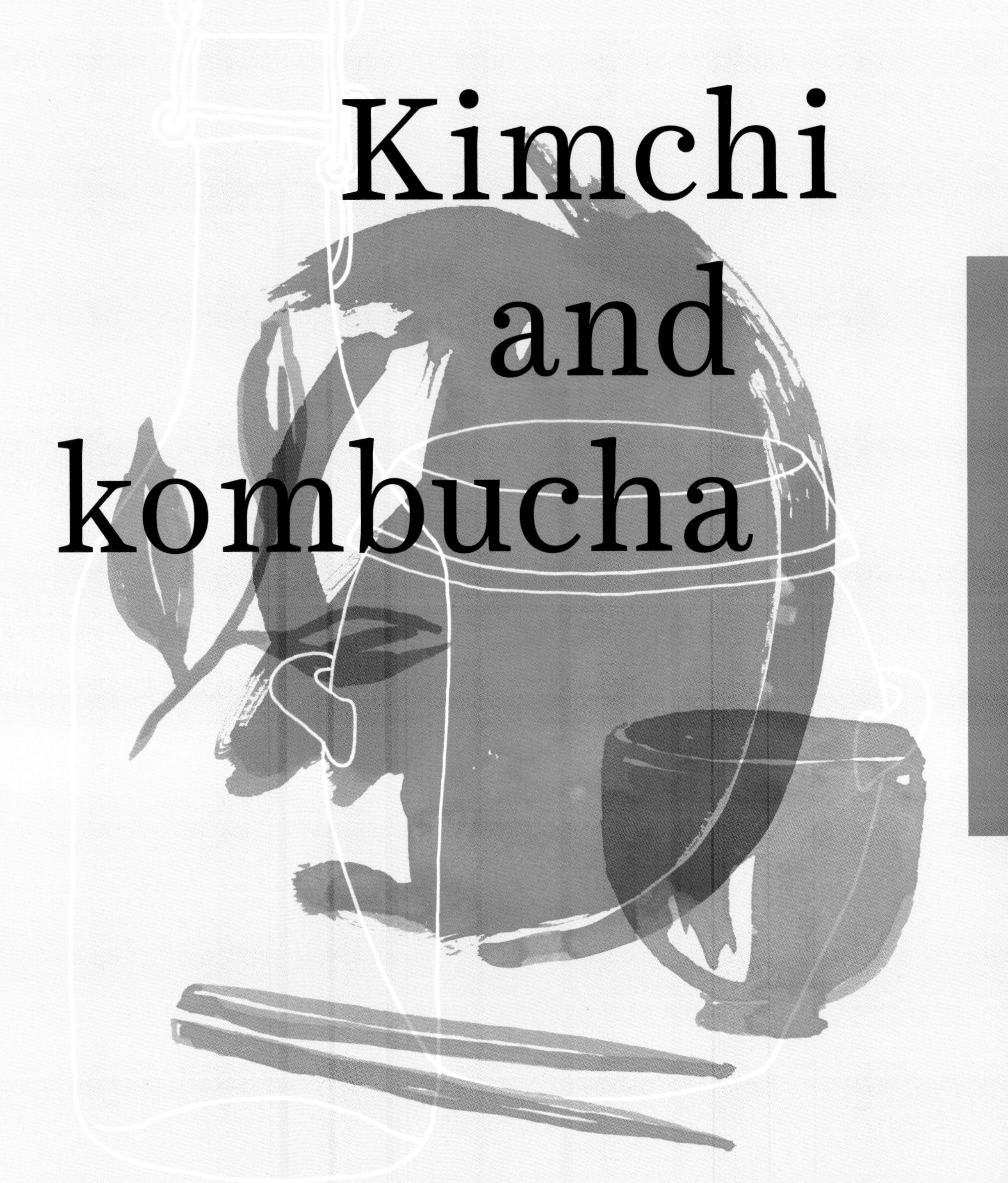

## *Korea's favorite health food*

Now that we know bacteria and fiber benefit our brain, the question is how to best get these so-called psychobiotics inside us. The answer is through the fermented foods kimchi and kombucha, both of which come from my second home country, Korea. Kimchi and kombucha consistently top the list of best probiotic foods, which is not hard to believe in light of the fact that as little as one gram of kimchi can contain 100 billion good bacteria. There's even a type of bacteria that has been named after kimchi—*Lactobacillus kimchi*.

As for kombucha, legend has it that kombucha was born when a Korean doctor, Dr. Kombu, healed the Japanese emperor over two thousand years ago from a serious disease with his magic tea—kombucha. These days, kombucha has reached the West where over half of all millennials in the United States drink kombucha. Even kimchi has become a hot favorite in hip celebrity restaurants around the world; these days, it's known as our new superfood.

I'll now bring you on a journey around the world of kimchi and kombucha, where I will go through everything from their nutritional values, health benefits, preparations, storage methods, and how to make the best of them for your health. Be prepared to learn everything you need to know about kimchi and kombucha, and of course I'll also share my best and tastiest recipes —all to strengthen your gut flora and brain.

## *Kimchi—the new superfood*

Kimchi is associated with Korea, and rightly so! If you say the word *kimchi* to a Korean person, you will see them positively shine. No other dish is more important for Koreans, who pretty much eat it with every meal. Did you know that people in Korea eat as much as 50 to 200 grams of kimchi per day? Kimchi contains 100 billion healthy bacteria per gram, which means up to several trillions of bacteria per day. Talk about daily gut-and-brain care! Additionally, South Koreans have the longest life span in the world, and some researchers believe it has to do with their large daily intake of kimchi.

So, what is kimchi? Kimchi is a traditional fermented side dish that is usually made from cabbage but can also be made from radishes, cucumber, and scallions. Vegetables are fermented together with spices such as chili, ginger, and garlic, and the finished kimchi has an umami taste—tart and strong at the same time and incredibly delicious with most foods. It is said that every Korean family has their own unique kimchi recipe, and it is pointless trying to gauge the amount of kimchi varieties that exist (even if the figure of two hundred is waved around). There are simply endless variants of kimchi in the country. And remember: even if kimchi is unique to Korea, the art of fermenting is an ancient way of preparing food in many different cultures, which lays the foundation of many of the good stuff in life.

**THE NUTRITIONAL VALUE OF KIMCHI**

Boasting an extremely low calorie content and high nutritional value (lactic acid bacteria, vitamins, minerals, fiber, organic acids, and so on), kimchi has grown in popularity in the West, especially among the health-conscious. With its extremely high psychobiotic bacterial content, kimchi has risen to the top of the list as our new probiotic superfood.

Kimchi is often highlighted as one of the world's healthiest dishes. Kimchi teems with trillions of healthy bacteria that are dominated by three genera—*Leuconostoc*, *Lactobacillus*, and *Weissella*, which are all kinds of lactic acid bacteria known to be important to our brain. Interestingly about 10 to 40 percent of the bacteria in kimchi are still unidentified. Kimchi is also low in calories,

**Soki Choi reflects on whether kimchi is the secret to a long life**

The whole world pricked up their ears when the highly regarded journal *The Lancet* recently published a 2017 report that revealed South Korea is the country whose citizens boast the longest life spans in the world. This means South Korea has surpassed Japan to become the "darkest blue" patch on earth. The big question everyone is asking is: What is their secret? Even if many factors contribute to South Korea's long life span, such as investment in health care, increased awareness of health, fewer traffic accidents, and the development of economic and social status, the healthy Korean food kimchi that everyone is talking about is at the helm of the debate. The amount of kimchi and other fermented foods (meaning fiber and beneficial bacteria) is not eaten in as high a volume anywhere else as it is in South Korea. For a long time, the Mediterranean diet was hailed as one of the healthiest, with olive oil as a superfood, but the focus has now moved eastward. The fermented foods kimchi, gochujang, soy, miso, and tofu have long been used in medicinal ways in South Korea, though of course it has not been until recently that the latest research on bacteria's central role to our health has demonstrated why kimchi, scientifically, can be considered the secret behind South Koreans' long lives.

with only 15 kcal per 100 grams. Kimchi is a good source of fiber (24 percent of kimchi's dry weight), several vitamins (A, B, C), minerals (phosphorus, iron, calcium, potassium), phytochemicals, amino acids, and small amounts of yeast. One portion of kimchi gives around 50 to 80 percent of the recommended daily dose of vitamin C. In addition, kimchi contains plenty of healthy organic acids (lactic acid, acetic acid, butyric acid, and so on) and antioxidants (flavonoids).

## The health benefits of kimchi

What does research say about kimchi's health benefits? With the increase in interest in probiotic food, articles on kimchi have exploded over the last few years. As with all fermented food, it can be hard to conduct proper studies. For example, it is impossible to standardize the subject as kimchi is living and constantly developing. Despite this, several positive health effects have been identified, and some of which coincide with chronic first-world diseases.

With its several trillion healthy bacteria, kimchi is the super probiotic. Add to that the high level of fiber in cabbage, which as a prebiotic fuels the growth of lactic acid bacteria, and you have a well-thought-out symbiosis. In a study from 2017, *L. plantarum* from kimchi was also shown to have high levels of an enzyme that breaks down lactose, which would be of interest to those with lactose intolerance. Simply put, this superfood should be very relevant to anyone with an imbalanced gut flora and/or who want to strengthen their brain health.

### DIABETES AND SUSTAINING WEIGHT

Studies on both animals and humans have shown that kimchi can have positive effects on diabetes. In a group of prediabetic patients, consuming 300 grams of kimchi per day over a month resulted in a lowering of resistance to insulin, as well as lower blood pressure.

Kimchi has even been shown to help keep your weight down. In a study from 2016, it was shown that a supplement of certain lactic acid bacteria (*L. sakei* and *L. plantarum*) that can be found in kimchi inhibited weight gain in animals that had been fed a diet rich in fat.

### CARDIOVASCULAR DISEASE

There are also grounds to believe that kimchi can lower cholesterol levels., though we don't know yet if it is due to the lactic acid bacteria *L. plantarum* and *L. sakei* or the yeast *Saccharomyces cerevisiaem*, both of which can be found in kimchi, though the latter in small amounts. Meanwhile, two studies on animals have shown that propionic acid in kimchi has positive effects on blood fats, which could reduce arteriosclerosis.

### IMMUNOLOGICAL DISEASES

Kimchi appears to have positive effects on our immune system. Above all, the lactic acid bacteria *L. plantarum*, which can be found in large amounts in kimchi, seems to have an effect on certain immune cells (see pp. 105–106). In 2018, researchers found lower levels of inflammation-producing substances in animals that had been fed with extracts of kimchi. This conclusion is also reflected in a large number of studies that show a clear link between lactic acid bacteria and their anti-inflammatory effect on the immune system.

#### INFLUENZA

There are strong grounds to believe that kimchi has antibacterial properties that can combat infections. Researchers have demonstrated that lactic acid bacteria from kimchi can prohibit the growth of harmful bacteria, such as *E. coli* (causes an upset stomach), salmonella, and *H. pylori* (causes stomach ulcers). All food that contains beneficial bacteria, especially fermented food, can potentially protect against infection when bacteria colonizes the gut—as long as they survive the stomach acids and bile in the gastrointestinal tract. Thankfully, researchers have shown that *L. plantarum* and other bacteria in kimchi manage to travel all the way to the intestines where they can combat harmful bacteria. Researchers have even found a new type of antibiotic that is produced by the *L. plantarum* in kimchi and that has been shown to be effective against antibiotic-resistant bacteria and viruses. Most South Koreans are convinced that the outbreak of bird flu (SARS) that affected many parts of Asia in 2003, but not South Korea, did not spread to the country thanks to kimchi! Another study from 2018 reported that animals who were given *L. plantarum* developed a greater resistance against the flu virus, further supporting the theory that kimchi has antipathogenic properties.

#### MENTAL HEALTH

With the recent huge interest in the role of gut bacteria in our mental health, many interesting studies have been produced on the gut-brain axis and the connection between gut bacteria and mental illness (see chapter 3)—with great news for kimchi. *L. brevis*, which can be found in kimchi, appears to have properties that could allow it to be used to prevent depression in the future, for example. Even with disorders like multiple sclerosis (MS) and Alzheimer's, studies on animals have reported positive results from an ingestion of *L. plantarum* and *L. brevis*, both found in copious amounts in kimchi. In animal studies, *L. planetarium* has been shown to affect levels of anxiety-like behavior. In addition, researchers have seen that both *L. brevis* and *L. buchneri* in kimchi can produce high levels of GABA, a substance that calms the activity in nerve cells. Medication that strengthens GABA's effect is used for anxiety and epilepsy, among other things. A study from 2016 showed that a supplement of *L. brevis* also helped patients with sleep problems.

Current, interesting research that looks at the link between gut bacteria and mental health is having promising results for kimchi and its lactic acid bacteria. Even if remaining research still needs to be conducted, I'm confident enough to suggest that eating kimchi will strengthen your brain (see p. 104).

## *Making kimchi*

Kimchi is mainly eaten as a side dish. In Korea, a meal without kimchi is considered incomplete. Other examples of fermented flavorings are soy sauce, miso, and gochujang (chili paste) that give Korean food a deep and complex umami taste. However, kimchi tops the list of Korean cuisine and food culture. Apart from accompanying all meals, kimchi is used in a range of dishes, such as stews, soups, pancakes, fried rice, nori rolls, and so on. Traditionally, a Korean women's ability to cook is judged by her ability to make kimchi. The younger generation, however, buys ready-made kimchi in stores. In this book, I share recipes for kimchi that are cheap and easy to throw together in your own kitchen; I've also included dishes that typically make use of kimchi (see recipes on pp. 140–154).

## The pantry

There is a saying that says kimchi can really be made from anything edible. As kimchi based on cabbage is the classic and most popular form of kimchi, like my recipes, but you choose from various ingredients as a base. One main rule is that they should be raw ingredients of the highest quality to get a really crispy, tangy, and delicious kimchi.

### CABBAGE

The cabbage that constitutes the base for kimchi is called *baechu* in Korean and is also known as Chinese cabbage, Korean cabbage, napa cabbage, and, of course, kimchi cabbage. Cabbage is



### Soki Choi reflects on kimchi as a "sacred food"

For Korean people, kimchi is more than food. It is considered to represent a uniquely Korean mentality, especially its characteristic red color from the chili, which is considered to mirror the spirit of the Korean people. During the Korean War, kimchi is said to have given the soldiers the strength and hope to carry on fighting. When South Korea was sending out their first astronaut, a special "space kimchi" was even prepared to accompany her into space. Even the miraculous economic development that South Korea has gone through over the last few decades is thought by some to be—no joke—thanks to kimchi. To convert a developing country to one of the world's strongest economies in such a short time required strength and stress like they had never experienced before, and many believe this was handled well thanks to kimchi. It might have sounded absurd a few years ago, but all this makes sense considering the latest research that shows the vast amounts of psychobiotic lactic acid bacteria in kimchi that can strengthen the brain and our resistance to stress.

### The origin of kimchi

Kimchi can be traced back to the period of the Three Kingdoms in Korea over two thousand years ago. Just like many other cultures in the world, Koreans developed different ways to preserve vegetables, such as salting, drying, and fermenting. Above all, the long and cold winters in Korea drove the development of kimchi during the months when it was difficult to find fresh vegetables. These days, kimchi is stored separately in chilled environments following tradition. Almost every Korean household has a separate fridge set to an optimal temperature to store kimchi.

The first kimchi was not actually made from cabbage but from wild onion, eggplant, bamboo shoots, and wild herbs that grew in the mountains. The first kimchi is believed to have been made by soaking these vegetables in a salty brine. Over time, kimchi developed into the lactic acid–rich cabbage we now know as kimchi. The fresh tartness from the lactic acid is a much-appreciated taste that, in addition to the heat from the chili, characterizes kimchi. Koreans have always classed kimchi as medicine, and in the old days as long as there was mature winter kimchi left in large clay pots buried underground, no Korean worried about their health. Today, we now know that it was vitamin C, organic acids, and plenty of healthy lactic acid bacteria that contributed to their health.

### Etymology

The word *kimchi* is believed to come from the Chinese word *chimchae*, which means "soaked vegetable." The word was later modernized to *jimchi* and later *kimchi*. That the word has its origins in Chinese is not surprising as Chinese characters were the only sign system used in Korea for a long time.

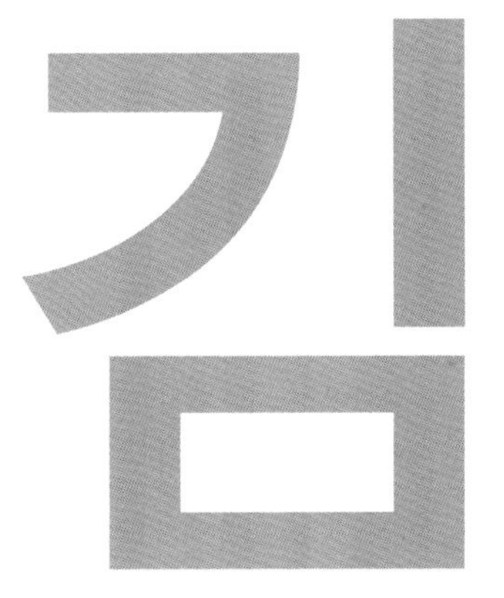


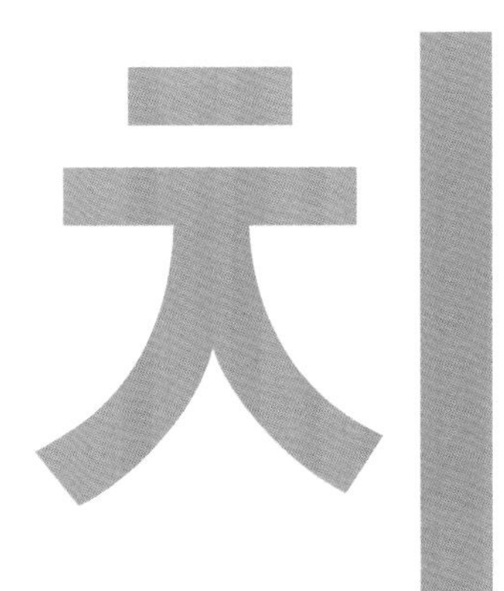

made up of around 95 percent water. The white parts of the leaves barely contain any vitamins; they are mostly located in the green parts. The perfect cabbage should therefore have lots of outer green leaves that should preferably be thin and lush.

#### SALT

Salt is vital to start the fermenting process. This is because salt starts off the lactic acid fermentation by allowing healthy, salt-hardy lactic acid bacteria to multiply while pushing out unwanted harmful bacteria that would otherwise cause decomposition and produce harmful substances, since harmful bacteria can't survive in a salty and acidic environment. Too little salt can therefore lead to unsuccessful fermentation with moldy, inedible cabbage that smells funky and rotten. The salt also reduces liquid content, which makes the raw product's texture crispy and crunchy rather than mushy. Salt also contributes to the taste, while extending the kimchi's use-by date. Coarse sea salt is ideal, but normal household salt also works as long as it doesn't contain iodine (iodine kills the good bacteria). Other salts should be avoided. If you use normal household salt (without iodine), you need to reduce the amount of salt as most recipes are written according to the use of sea salt—otherwise, the kimchi will be too salty.

#### GARLIC

Garlic contains many vitamins, which keep blood lipids balanced and reduce high blood pressure. Some people struggle with the strong taste of garlic, which comes from allyl sulfide, but garlic is a really important ingredient when making kimchi. The fermentation process and kimchi's final bacterial constitution is greatly affected by garlic.

#### GINGER

Fresh ginger, which is rich in minerals, is also an obligatory ingredient in kimchi. The typical ginger taste comes from gingerol and shogaol, and apart from contributing a lovely spicy flavor, it also provides positive effects and is said to reduce inflammation and strengthen the immune system.

#### GOCHUGARU

Another necessary ingredient for kimchi is gochugaru—red chili flakes that are made from sun-dried chili pepper. Gochugaru has a texture that is in between flakes and powder, and the taste is sweet, soft, full-bodied, and somewhat smoky with a distinctive heat that is also not too strong. There is no way you can swap gochugaru for cayenne, sambal oelek, or any other variety of red chili pepper; it just won't be kimchi. Gochugaru can easily be found in Asian grocery stores or online. Remember: there are different types of gochugaru with a range of chili heats. Many prefer the milder version of gochugaru. Gochugaru is what makes kimchi red, so use more if you want your kimchi redder. It is important that the gochugaru is not finely ground, as that won't make kimchi. After you open a package of gochugaru, keep it in the freezer, tightly sealed, so it will stay fresh longer.

**Soki Choi reflects on salt and sugar in healthy kimchi**

Salt is a fundamental part of kimchi's fermentation process, stimulating the growth of healthy lactic acid bacteria and organic acids, which in turn prevent mold and harmful bacteria from developing. This is why there is such a low risk of getting an infection or food poisoning from fermented food like kimchi—if you use enough salt. Don't do what my friend once did—she used too little salt because she thought it would make the kimchi healthier, but instead turned it moldy and inedible! The same goes with sugar, which has a fermentation function and basically disappears during the process. The use of fermented fish sauce (unless you are vegan) and garlic also play an important role. In other worlds, all the ingredients used to make kimchi have a central function in the fermentation process, so respect it and follow the recipes exactly—especially in the beginning—and you will get tasty and healthy kimchi. Good luck!

**FISH SAUCE**

Traditionally made kimchi typically has a fishy smell because some type of fermented fish sauce or salty, fermented tiny shrimps, sardines, octopus, oysters, or anchovies are used. The fermented fish sauce adds the amino acid glutamic acid, which gives kimchi its sought-after and hard-to-describe taste of umami. Umami is the fifth taste that gives a deep and rich savory taste of broth. Umami can be found in soy, miso, and seaweed. Umami, which in Japanese means "good taste," strengthens flavor profiles and makes the mouth water. In addition to contributing an umami taste, the fermented fish sauce kick-starts the fermentation process. But even if most Koreans consider fermented fish sauce to be vital in the preparation of kimchi, you can make kimchi without fish sauce if you are vegan, vegetarian, or allergic to fish or shellfish—simply replace the fish sauce with salt (1 tablespoon of fish sauce is equivalent to 1 teaspoon of salt).

## The ABCs of kimchi

Despite the two-thousand-year history of kimchi and its place in myths and legends, it is not difficult to actually make it. You do not need advanced equipment or tools—just your hands and a knife. The only basic rule is that kimchi requires time and patience; it is not fast food but rather prefers to develop in peace. The fermentation period takes usually about a week, but kimchi can be ready to eat after just a few days. Preparing classic kimchi can be summarized in three steps (for more details, see the recipes on pp. 140–154).

#### A. PICKLING

Salt a cabbage and place it in a salty brine. Leave for a few hours, preferably overnight. Rinse the leaves in cold water to remove excess salt.

#### B. FLAVORING

Prepare a kimchi filling. The ingredients vary by recipe but generally contain garlic, ginger, fish sauce, leek, and gochugaru. Spread some kimchi filling on each leaf and then pack the cabbage tightly in a large glass jar with a tightly sealed lid.

#### C. FERMENTING

Fermenting begins by letting the sealed jar of kimchi stand in room temperature for the first twenty-four hours. Lactic acid bacteria prefer this environment and will quickly multiply. Then, place the kimchi jar in the fridge and allow the fermentation process to continue until the kimchi is ready to eat.

The amount of days required to let the kimchi sit vary, depending on the recipe, temperature, and personal taste. Some types of kimchi, like cucumber kimchi, tastes best after a short time, while others develop deeper and more complex tastes the longer you let them ferment. A general rule of thumb is that the lower the temperature, the longer fermentation takes. It is important not to open the jar during the process—the less oxygen you let in, the greater your chance of getting perfect kimchi. You will often see small bubbles from carbonation appear, building up pressure in the jar. If you use a plastic jar, the jar might start to bulge out a bit, which is perfectly normal.

After four to five days, you can open the jar and do a taste test. Start by smelling—it should smell tangy and fresh with clear notes of kimchi filling. When it is time to taste it, use a clean fork—do *not* use your hands as it can disturb the lactic acid bacteria in kimchi.

#### THE MOST COMMON BEGINNER'S MISTAKE

It is difficult to completely fail with kimchi, even if it does not always turn out optimal, taste-wise. The most common beginner's mistake is that too little salt is used, which would allow mold to appear. You also want to take note to avoid too much yeast from forming, which makes the kimchi softer and sourer over the fermentation period. The amount of yeast from saccharomyces in the kimchi increases especially at the end of fermentation, which is usually around thirty days of being stored in the fridge. The levels of health-promoting *L. plantarum* and *L. brevis* will also increase toward the end of fermentation, so if you want the highest levels of lactic acid bacteria, "harvest" the kimchi just before it gets too ripe.

## Optimizing kimchi

The following tips for optimizing kimchi are not necessary for when you make kimchi at home. These bonus tips are more for kimchi nerds who, like scientists in research laboratories, wish to experiment with and optimize their kimchi.

#### STARTER LIQUID

Kimchi usually ferments without a starter liquid or other bacterial cultures, but researchers have begun to prepare probiotic "kimchi starters" with different combinations of lactic acid bacteria. Starter liquids have been shown to increase the chances of successful fermentation, allowing the process to happen quicker. A better taste and health benefits can result from these customized "kimchi starters." A tried-and-tested traditional housewife trick is to add a little liquid from an earlier fermentation of kimchi, which increases the chances of a successful result. It is the exact same method as when you prepare kombucha or sourdough bread.

**Tips:**
When the kimchi has fermented too much, it can be used as an ingredient in hot or cooked dishes such as kimchi stew (see p. 153), where all the bacteria will disappear in the cooking process, but the kimchi will still contribute a fantastic taste and tartness for die-hard kimchi fans.

#### FERMENTATION TIME

If you want to optimize the health effects of kimchi, experiment with its fermentation times. The amount of bacteria in kimchi increases a hundredfold during the fermentation period, reaching its peak after twelve to eighteen days at 40 degrees Fahrenheit (fridge temperature) and maintaining this level for at least twenty-nine days of fermentation (one month). If you want to get the probiotic *Lactococcus lactis*, the kimchi has to have an even longer fermentation period.

#### TEMPERATURE

The lower the temperature, the longer it takes for kimchi to ferment to reach an optimal taste, longevity, and the ideal pH level of around 4.5. In lower temperatures (40 to 48 degrees), it takes around four weeks for kimchi to be ready to eat. If you ferment kimchi at room temperature (68 to 71.5 degrees) it takes around another three days. Then the kimchi has to remain chilled in the fridge (below 46 degrees). Interestingly, the doubling of vitamin C and B are also reached at cold fermentation (40 degrees) after two to three weeks, before the levels start to drop.

#### BACTERIA

In the beginning of the process, the bacteria *Leuconostoc mesenteroides* dominates to kick-start fermentation. As the fermenting continues, lactic acids from the species *Lactobacillus* increase. The amount of weissella bacteria is fairly stable during the whole fermenting process. The bacteria that can be found in each individual ingredient also affect kimchi's final bacterial constitution. Research shows that while cabbage doesn't have a big effect on fermentation, it is garlic that mainly contributes to the increase of lactic acid bacteria—the more garlic that is used, the more lactic acid bacteria there is. In addition, kimchi with chili pepper features more bacteria from the *Weissella* species and less from the *Leuconostoc* and *Lactobacillus* species when compared to kimchi without. By choosing the raw ingredients, you can control the mix of bacteria in your kimchi.

## *Kombucha—a bubbly probiotic*

In recent years, kombucha has risen to the top as the new *cool* drink. Thanks to its probiotic reputation, it has become very popular among celebrities and influencers in the United States. In New York and Los Angeles, kombucha is commonly drunk both at the bar as well as after a yoga session. If you google kombucha, you will get more than 13 million hits. In Sweden, *kombucha* became an official word in 2017's list of new and popular words, demonstrating that kombucha is here to stay. But what is it? Kombucha is a slightly carbonated and tangy drink that is packed full of lovely bacteria. The mythical kombucha hails from Korea and is brewed from tea and bacterial cultures (SCOBY, which stands for symbiotic culture of bacteria and yeast). Kombucha has long belonged to the hippy culture but has since been hijacked by trendy, health-conscious millennials who have made kombucha their new, favorite drink instead of soda and juice. Kombucha is also vegan, raw, and living, making it a popular drink among organic and ethically conscious consumers. In other words, kombucha is of its time, and the public's growing interest in it over the last few years has even resulted in an increase in the amount of scientific articles on the subject. Research reports that kombucha contains plenty of lactic acid bacteria and organic acids that have been shown to contribute to a healthier gut flora and a stronger brain.

#### THE HEALTH EFFECTS OF KOMBUCHA

Kombucha has been hailed as a miracle elixir, and its list of beneficial effects on our health seems almost endless. It has been suggested that kombucha can do everything from eliminating gray hair and increasing sexual appetite to enhancing vision and combating the aging process.

Even if the field of research is fairly young and limited, the first recognizable health benefits are starting to emerge. So far, studies on animals show that kombucha's positive health effects are mainly due to its composition of healthy organic acids and antioxidants. Here are some of its preliminary health benefits: combats free radicals, kills off harmful bacteria (great for upset stomachs), detoxifies, protects the liver, lowers cholesterol, thins blood, improves digestion, and prevents cancer, diabetes, and asthma.

The fact that different substances in kombucha are beneficial for different health conditions show its ability to treat our body as a whole system, rather than treating a specific organ.

As I showed in the bacterial guide in chapter 4, there are mainly two bacterial genera that have been systematically investigated and that have shown to have psychobiotic properties—*Lactobacillus* and *Bifidobacterium*. The good news is that studies show that both lactobacillus and bifidobacterium are present in kombucha (even if the levels vary depending on the quality of SCOBY).

Remember that kombucha is a living ecosystem that can vary greatly from brew to brew. Even as we wait for more research to be conducted, you can still start to consume kombucha to strengthen your gut flora, brain, and mental health.

### THE NUTRITIONAL VALUE OF KOMBUCHA

Kombucha contains a lot of biochemical substances and living bacteria. Above all, the metabolite organic acid dominates kombucha. There is still a lot more research that needs to be done, but luckily new discoveries are being reported all the time.

Let's now take a closer look at the larger substances that have so far been discovered in kombucha.

### AMINO ACIDS

The kombucha culture SCOBY contains nine essential amino acids, which actually makes it a complete protein. (Protein is needed for the muscles, immune system, and metabolism to work correctly.) As a result, some people even eat SCOBY for a health boost! The amount of amino acids increases with the fermentation process—in one study, the highest level was reached after twenty-one days of fermentation with black tea.

### ORGANIC ACIDS

When the body builds and sustains functions such as creating body tissue, healing sores, and detoxing medication and toxins, it needs organic acids. The main acids that are produced when brewing kombucha are acetic acid, lactic acid, gluconic acid, and glucuronic acid. Even the anti-inflammatory butyric acid, which has been shown to have a positive effect on the brain and mental health (see p. 44), is found in kombucha.

### BACTERIA

Kombucha is teeming with bacteria—one milliliter of kombucha contains around half a million bacteria after one to two weeks of fermentation. The bacterial species that dominates kombucha is *Gluconacetobacter*, which produces the healthy acids gluconic acid and glucuronic acid. Gluconacetobacter is the main contributor to the production of cellulose (fiber) and therefore new kombucha cultures.

In addition, the bacterial types vary a lot depending on which SCOBY the kombucha is brewed with. Kombucha that has come into contact with dirt while brewing can lead to a reduced level of healthy lactic acid bacteria, so it is really important to keep any contaminants away when brewing.

### POLYPHENOLS

Polyphenols are a strong antioxidant that give fruit and vegetables their color, odor, and taste. There are over eight thousand polyphenols and the most well-known type is flavonoids, which can be found in abundance in green and black tea (and even red wine). The flavonoids in tea give kombucha its antioxidant and antibacterial properties. Polyphenols are known for their preventative effects against diseases like cancer, cardiovascular disease, and diabetes, while tea has long been prescribed as a toxic-free, natural, and safe alternative or supplement to medicine. New studies show that kombucha brewed with black tea drastically increases polyphenols. What is more exciting is that kombucha is also a source of new polyphenols that were not originally in the tea.

#### YEASTS

The yeast content in kombucha varies greatly between different SCOBY and goes through a transformation during fermentation. There doesn't seem to be a specific type that can be found in all kombucha; rather the yeast content seems to be influenced by the origin of the SCOBY and which yeasts can be found in that part of the world where the SCOBY comes from. Even if research on the probiotic effects of yeasts are few and far between, preliminary studies point to the fact that some types of yeast can contribute to good health. A new study from 2018, for example, shows that the yeast *Saccharomyces cerevisiae*, which is commonly found in kombucha, has an effect of lowering cholesterol on mice and cell cultures.

#### VITAMINS AND MINERALS

Kombucha is rich in vitamins B, B1, B2, B6, B12, and B9 (folic acid), as well as vitamin C. The B vitamins, which play an essential role in a cell's metabolic process, are produced when the yeast in kombucha breaks down the sugar. Research shows that fermentation increases the amount of vitamin B, where a study found around 200 percent more vitamin B in kombucha when compared to normal tea. Even levels of vitamin C increase during fermentation.

#### ALCOHOL

In all processes of fermentation, traces of alcohol naturally occur as a by-product. Kombucha that is brewed at home usually contains 0.2 to 0.5 percent, which is low enough to be classed as alcohol-free. Exactly how much alcohol that is produced in kombucha depends on several factors, such as the constitution of the yeast in the kombucha culture, the temperature, and amount of sugar. Many studies have shown that small amounts of alcohol have blood-thinning effects. Normal homebrewed kombucha seldom reaches over 2 percent of alcohol, but if you want to raise or lower the alcohol level, you can adjust the temperature, yeast, and/or sugar in different ways.



## *Making kombucha*

To start your kombucha brew, you need to do a bit of prep. Once you've started, it is easy to carry on with the brewing. Here is what you'll need for the raw ingredients and equipment, as well as instructions. You can also find more detailed recipes in the book (pp. 158–159).

#### THE PANTRY

Before you start to make your own kombucha, it might be useful if you know someone who regularly brews kombucha so you can use their leftover starter liquid or SCOBY, since brewing kombucha usually produces more starter liquid and SCOBY than needed. Otherwise, you can buy SCOBY on the Internet. Once the starter liquid (kombucha) and SCOBY have been procured, things get easier as all you'll need next is water, tea leaves, and a little bit of sugar to begin brewing your kombucha.

**SCOBY AND STARTER LIQUID**

To brew kombucha, you need something called SCOBY as well as a really sour starter liquid. SCOBY, which stands for *symbiotic culture of bacteria and yeast*, is the actual kombucha culture. SCOBY is also loosely known as *kombucha mushroom*, *tea fungus*, or *Volga mushroom* since it looks like a smooth white mushroom. In reality, SCOBY is a thick carpet of biofilm mainly consisting of the fiber cellulose that stimulates and feeds millions of bacteria in the kombucha. In this prebiotic SCOBY, plenty of bacteria live and flourish. Using SCOBY together with the starter liquid drives the fermenting process forward. The term SCOBY was coined in 1996 in order to differentiate the kombucha culture from the starter liquid.

The starter liquid is a mature kombucha liquid that, together with the SCOBY, kick-starts the fermentation of the tea. A strong starter liquid should be really sour and at least two weeks old, but preferably even older between four to six weeks, otherwise there is a risk of getting a diluted kombucha without any power to ferment. The first time you brew kombucha at home, it is worth ordering SCOBY and starter liquid (the SCOBY is always in the starter liquid) through a reputable seller whom you can easily find on the Internet. Be sure that the order contains fresh SCOBY (absolutely not dried or frozen) and at least 0.8 cups of really sour starter liquid. Remember that the constitution of the bacteria and yeast vary between different types of SCOBY. Many SCOBY sellers have a table of contents that list which bacteria their SCOBY consists of. A good alternative is getting SCOBY and starter liquid from someone you know who already makes kombucha. After your first brew, you'll never have to get any more SCOBY or starter liquid as continuous brewing of kombucha generates new SCOBY and starter liquid that you can then share with others.

**The origin of kombucha**

Kombucha has probably been drunk for several thousands of years in East Asia, but its first documented use can be traced back to a Korean doctor by the name of Dr. Kombu around 220 BC. Buddhist texts give a detailed description on how the Japanese emperor Ingiyo, who suffered from digestive problems, called on Dr. Kombu from the Silla kingdom (now Korea). Dr. Kombu brought with him some fermented tea from Korea and managed to cure the Japanese emperor's stomach problems. Tea is called *cha* in Korean and Japanese, as well as several Indian and Chinese languages. *Kombucha* can therefore be translated to "Dr. Kombu's tea."

That kombucha has its origins in Korea is not strange in light of the country's long tradition of drinking tea and using fermentation in the kitchen.

#### TEA LEAVES

Tea contributes many important substances that make the production of kombucha possible. The traditional and original way to produce kombucha was to brew it using black tea, but these days it is also popular to use green tea or a mix of black and green. Black tea is completely oxidized and has more caffeine/theine than other types of tea; meanwhile green tea is not completely oxidized and its leaves are steamed, which makes it rich in polyphenols (see p. 125). You can also try to make kombucha with white tea, which, I believe, is the healthiest and most delicious tea!

It doesn't really matter which type of tea you use to make kombucha, but one thing worth noting is that the temperature of the water and how long to steep the tea for will vary among tea types. Some kombucha fanatics believe you should use loose black tea without any flavor—so, for example, you should not use Earl Grey because of its bergamot oils. There is no scientific basis that tea bags or flavored tea won't work—as long as they don't contain artificial



### Soki Choi reflects on kombucha as a "sacred food"

Kombucha has a reputation of doing everything, from preventing cancer, diabetes, rheumatism, aging, and obesity to improving hair, skin, and nails. Its appeal has spread to health-conscious consumers in recent years, and it has, along with its health benefits, also brought with it a surprising lifestyle philosophy. Once you start brewing kombucha at home, the mother culture continuously creates new baby cultures, introducing a new life cycle into our daily lives. These new baby cultures also prompt you to share them with other people (just like the philosophy of making sourdough) so they, too, can start brewing their own healthy kombucha for themselves and others. In addition, this continuous cycle of brewing and drinking nurtures your gut flora and health. Fermenting kombucha takes time, allowing you to practice your patience—and it's not hard! Personally, for me, kombucha provides a link to an ancient Asian food wisdom that has been passed down through generations, from country to country, and that has survived for thousands of years. I call that sacred food!

chemicals that can kill bacteria. Research also shows that you can brew healthy kombucha from leaves other than tea leaves (for example, eucalyptus or oak leaves), which gives the kombucha a different biochemical profile.

#### SUGAR

Many people worry that sugar is used in preparing kombucha, but note that the sugar is needed to feed the kombucha culture SCOBY with nutrients, if not it will die. The sugar is eventually eaten up by the yeast during the fermentation process (just like the process of making wine), which converts the sugar to organic acids and other healthy substances. This means that only a small amount of sugar is left in the finished kombucha. The longer it ferments, the less sugar there will be and the sourer the kombucha. The recommended amount of sugar is usually 50 to 100 grams per 2 pints of kombucha liquid. Even if a host of factors affect the sugar level, you can roughly say that tea with an initial sugar level of 50 grams per 2 pints per is roughly 1 to 2.5 grams of sugar per 0.4 cups of finished kombucha. In comparison, fruit juice contains 11 grams of sugar per 0.4 cup of juice. It is worth noting that sugar in finished kombucha turns to glucose and fructose, which has a lower glycemic index than normal sugar, making kombucha suitable for people with diabetes. Using too little sugar, however (less than 30 grams per 2 pints), has been shown to make the kombucha so weak and nutrient-poor that it doesn't have the energy to start the fermenting process or produce strong living SCOBY. In other words, don't be afraid of using sugar in a kombucha recipe—it is not meant to feed you but rather to feed the bacteria so they can produce healthy substances. The best types of sugar to use are usually regular sugar or raw sugar. Essentially, SCOBY is dependent on being fed with nutrients and energy in the form of sweet, tepid tea in order to produce the healthy concoction in finished kombucha.

**Tips:**
After the basic brew, many people choose to flavor and carbonize the kombucha by adding fruit or juice, which contains natural sugars. This principle is the same as with brewing beer—the more sugar you add, the more carbon is produced.

### Equipment

#### GLASS JAR

To make a basic kombucha brew, a large, clean glass jar is the best and most common vessel to brew in. Even a good-quality stainless steel container should work to ferment kombucha in, but avoid metals like brass, iron, and aluminum as they can't handle the kombucha's low pH levels—the acids may dissolve the metal, allowing it to leak into the kombucha.

#### FABRIC

A clean tea towel or large piece of fabric, preferably cotton, is needed to cover the glass jar during the first brew. The fabric has two main functions. First, it protects the kombucha against dust, spores, fruit flies, and other potential contaminants. This is why it is important that the fabric is not too porous so contaminants can't pass through. An elastic band that is secured around the fabric and glass jar will keep it in place. Second, the fabric should allow fresh air to seep through to provide oxygen to the SCOBY so that respiration, which is vital for the first basic brew, can take place. This is why the fabric can't be too dense as oxygen needs to pass through. For oxygenation to reach optimal levels, the top of the glass jar should be as wide as possible and not too narrow.

**BOTTLES**

For the second stage of fermentation, during which you flavor and bottle the kombucha, you need a bunch of bottles to fill the kombucha with. The bottles need to be airtight to allow carbonation, but since the pressure can build up, some people prefer using plastic bottles, making sure the plastic is safe for food. Personally, I prefer glass bottles and have never experienced an exploding bottle. Make sure that the lid or cork doesn't contain metal that can oxidize—if

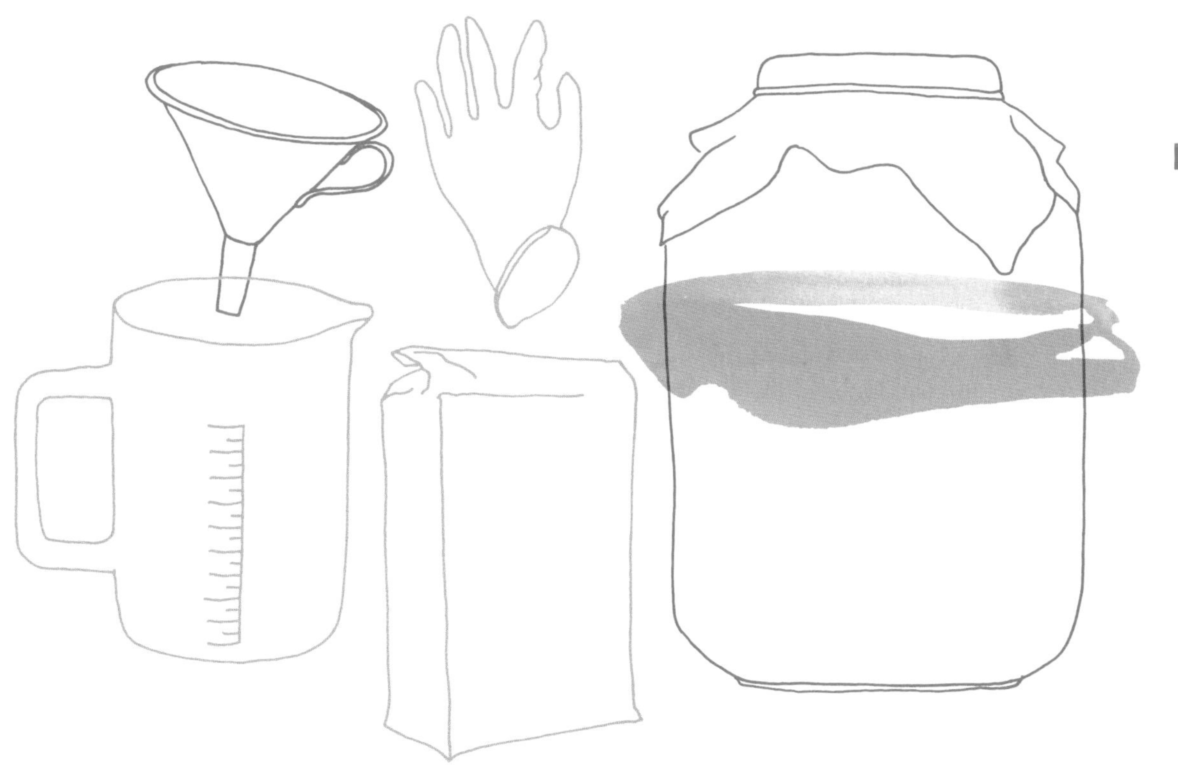

any rust appears around the lid, you'll have to throw the kombucha away.

**OTHER TOOLS**

- **Plastic gloves:** Cleanliness is first and foremost when handling SCOBY and kombucha. Even if it should be enough to simply wash your hands in soap and hot water, you can use extra protection with plastic gloves.
- **Straws:** If your glass jar doesn't have a tap to pour the kombucha out of, it is worth getting a bunch of plastic straws so you can taste the kombucha during the fermentation process without coming into contact with the drink.
- **Labels:** In my experience, it is hard to recall when you started the first brew if you don't write the date clearly on a label or directly onto the glass jar. Labeling makes it easier to know when you need to test it and when to start flavoring and bottling it.
- **Funnel and sieve:** When pouring the kombucha into glass bottles, it really helps to use a funnel; otherwise the process can get rather wet. A large, dense sieve can also help to remove tea leaves after the first basic brew and even after the second fermentation when you may need to remove bits of fruit and berries that can easily turn pale and soggy.

## The ABCs of kombucha

Kombucha is a constantly changing biomass just like gut flora, which means that the kombucha will vary each time. Many factors, such as the type of tea, amount of sugar, temperature, and fermentation time will affect how the kombucha develops and tastes. Even if you follow a recipe to a T, the kombucha will taste different each time, even between brews, since the kombucha culture (SCOBY) and starter liquid that is reused from the first brew will have a different bacteria content, yeast, and acids. A good kombucha has a fresh and sweet-sour aroma that leans slightly toward the taste of vinegar. Kombucha also changes color and gets lighter during the brewing process.

Kombucha is a living drink that can't be completely controlled, which also gives it personality. Just like in life, kombucha has an unpredictable side that invites you to dare to experiment, let go, and trust the process.

## The basic brew

If there is one basic rule you need to remember when making kombucha, it is cleanliness. As SCOBY is a living biomass containing bacteria and yeast, I can't stress enough how important hygiene is. Wash your hands carefully and for a long time with normal soap in warm water. Wash all the containers and equipment that you plan to use in washing liquid and hot water. Just avoid antiseptic soap and washing liquid that can kill the bacteria in the SCOBY and starter liquid. Then, get going! If you don't have any further biochemical interest in the process of fermentation or the mix of bacteria and yeast in your kombucha, it can be very simple to make your own kombucha. The whole process can be summarized in three simple steps (see the basic recipe on pp. 158–159):

### Soki Choi's tips: White tea is the healthiest and tastes the best

After having tasted my way through countless types of kombuchas and experimented with different types of tea, I'm stuck on white tea. White tea is made from the youngest and most delicate leaves that are covered in fine white hairs and harvested during a brief period in the year. This is why white tea is considered the queen of all teas. The leaves don't oxidize but go through a careful drying process to protect its delicate taste and content. This means that white tea has the highest level of antioxidants of all tea types, making white tea the healthiest. Most of all, it is the taste that makes white tea my favorite to use when brewing kombucha. White tea has a mild and somewhat sweet taste that is not as bitter as other types of tea.



**A. PREPARE SWEET, TEPID TEA**

Boil water, add some tea leaves/tea bags and sugar, and leave to cool down.

**B. ADD SCOBY AND STARTER LIQUID**

Pour the sweet tea into a glass jar, then add the SCOBY and finally the starter liquid.

**C. LET SIT AND WAIT A WEEK**

Secure a piece of fabric on top and leave the glass jar undisturbed for a week in room temperature.

After a week, do a taste test with a straw to see if you like the flavor. If you want a tangier kombucha, leave it to ferment for a few more days. When you are satisfied, you can "harvest" the basic kombucha, bottle it, and place in the fridge. It is now ready to drink naturally as-is, which is the traditional way of consuming kombucha. You can also choose to flavor the brew and let the kombucha go through a second fermentation process (see below).

A new daughter-SCOBY develops during the first fermentation. It looks like a thin white membrane and it always lies at the top of the brew. You can reuse this to make a new batch of basic brew or give to a friend who wants to make kombucha.

**FLAVORING AND CARBONATING (OPTIONAL)**

Flavoring kombucha is a modern trend. This stage of the preparation is what many people enjoy the most since it allows them to be most creative. What can you flavor kombucha with? You can use anything from fresh, frozen, or dried fruit and berries to jams, syrups, and juice, as long as the don't contain artificial additives. I have shared some of my favorite flavorings in my recipes (p. 159), but in reality the only limit is your imagination.

So, how do you flavor kombucha? Get a bunch of clean bottles and add in your flavor of choice (I usually fill about one-fifth of the bottle). Then, fill it all the way to the top with ready kombucha from the first fermentation. It's important that there be hardly any air left in the bottle and that the lid or cork is secured on tight so that carbon dioxide from the carbonation process can't seep out. When you add flavor to the second brew, the yeast wakes up and starts to turn the sugar in the fruit or juice into carbon dioxide, which forces the process of carbonation. Sometimes this happens so fast that it is worth opening the bottles once a day to avoid accidents—it is smart to always open kombucha bottles over the sink! If you want to reduce the amount of fizz, put them in the fridge as this reduces the yeast's production of carbon dioxide. Another way to reduce carbonation is to lessen the amount of added sugar by using less fruit, berries, juice, etc. You can also try to filter the yeast away with a sieve or a nut bag before you bottle the kombucha.

In traditional brews, very little or no carbon is created, and the drink is just as healthy when enjoyed with very little fizz. However, if your intention is to create fizz, make sure you have enough yeast in the bottles when you bottle the drink. Feed the yeast with sugar either in the form of sweet fruits or juice, which typically has more sugar than, say, berries; some also cheat by adding regular sugar. Then seal the bottles tight and leave them at room temperature for one to five days. The number of days depends on a range of factors, such as the yeast and sugar levels in your specific choice of flavor, the temperature, and so on. The cooler the temperature, the longer the bottles need to stand. When you feel that a sufficient amount of carbon has built up, they are ready to drink and you can then store the bottles in the fridge.

## Optimizing your kombucha

These are tips for those who have been brewing kombucha for a while and want to take it to the next level!

#### TEMPERATURE AND STORAGE

Most people ferment at room temperature (68 to 71.5 degrees), but the range of temperatures recommended for fermenting kombucha is 68 to 86 degrees and the optimal temperature is considered to be 78.5 to 80.5 degrees.

If you brew in a temperature that is too low (less than 68 degrees), the kombucha will be weak and slushy with an increased risk of mold. Many kombucha experts therefore prefer fermenting in an environment slightly warmer than room temperature (73.5 to 80.5 degrees) to speed up the fermentation and production of carbon.

As this optimal temperature is somewhat warmer than room temperature, the warm top of the fridge is a popular storage place among many kombucha makers. Many people store their kombucha in the pantry, though darkness is not necessary. Wherever you store your kombucha, it is important for air to be flowing through. My advice is to ferment at normal room temperature in a suitable half-shaded area in the kitchen.

When the basic brew and any flavoring step is complete, the bottled kombucha is stored in the fridge, which almost stops the fermentation process. If the kombucha is handled and stored properly, it will last for as long as you are willing to drink it. Fermentation continues very slowly even in the fridge, which means the kombucha will get sourer over time, finally turning into vinegar. Kombucha vinegar can be drunk like a "shrub" (a strong shot) or used for salad dressings (see p. 167).

#### FERMENTATION TIME

Fermentation time depends on several factors, such as temperature, sugar levels, type of tea, taste preference, and the amount of liquid. It is almost impossible to provide the perfect fermentation time; you simply have to test your way there based on your unique kombucha brew. A general guideline is seven to twelve days.

Bacterial diversity reaches its peak after seven days of fermentation and starts to reduce after this period. Studies have shown that a week's worth of fermentation leads to a shift of the dominant yeast from candida to lachancea. The longer fermentation continues, the better kombucha is able to clear up free radicals. probably due to the increase in antioxidant flavonoids. And as I've mentioned, the level of organic acids increases the longer fermentation occurs.

#### PH VALUE

The tartness of the kombucha depends on your taste preference (whenever you choose to stop the fermentation process). Some prefer their kombucha a bit sourer, with the taste leaning toward a vinegary profile, while others prefer a sweeter variant. The general pH range thought to be ideal for kombucha is 2.5 to 3.5; a lower pH level gives a sourer drink. Personally, I have found that a pH level of 3 provides the perfect balance between sweet and sour, but you need to do your own experimentation. The main rule is that the longer it ferments, the sourer it becomes. After three to five days, the pH value will have already sunk to under 3.5. After three to four weeks of fermentation, the pH value will reach 2 to 2.5, which is equivalent to the values in lemon or tomato juice. An increased level of sourness means that there is also an increased amount of healthy organic acids. This is why it is good to pour the starter liquid in last when working on a basic brew—adding it on top of the kombucha culture (SCOBY) acts as an extra protection against harmful bacteria and substances.

If you want to follow the development of pH levels in your kombucha, you can get a pH meter to help, but often your tongue is enough to taste for the level of tanginess.

#### MOLD

If you follow the recipe to a T, are careful with hygiene, and use high-quality products, it is unlikely that your kombucha will develop mold. If this should happen in any case, you'll need to throw the whole lot away and start again. Don't save anything, even the kombucha liquid. The whole SCOBY and any new SCOBY will have to be thrown out. When you are checking for mold, make sure it really is mold that you see. Many newbies mistake the brown-colored yeast that grows and floats around or seeps into the SCOBY and creates dark patches as mold. Even remnants of tea leaves can get stuck in the SCOBY and create lumps or patches that can be mistaken for mold. Mold looks exactly like it does on other foods—white, green, blue, or black—and it is dry and coarse. The mold in kombucha is always found on top of the SCOBY, and never underneath it or in the liquid. Below is a list of factors that can cause mold.

- **Low temperature:** brewing at a low temperature makes the bacteria slow, which can cause the kombucha not to sour fast enough.
- **Too little starter liquid:** one of the most common reasons behind moud is that not enough starter liquid is used or that it is too weak.
- **Air pollutants:** mold spores are invisible and can lie dormant in the surrounding area. In addition, some houseplants release pollen that can transport mold spores. In this case, make sure to brew in a separate room away from plants.
- **Contaminated ingredients:** tea can be sprayed with pesticides or other chemicals that have a negative impact on the SCOBY.

Even water can be contaminated, which can harm the SCOBY and cause mold. That's why you need to make sure the ingredients are of the highest quality.

Extreme damp: damp feeds certain bacteria and types of yeasts that are harmful to the SCOBY and can cause mold. If you find yourself in a very damp environment, it is worth using a fan around the brewing process.

The most vulnerable time during the brewing is the first three to four days when beneficial bacteria and yeast types have not yet colonized the kombucha enough to resist potential intruders such as mold spores. It is extra important to protect the brew against mold and other contaminants at the beginning of the brewing process. First, the starter liquid needs to be really mature and sour (at least four to six weeks); newly brewed kombucha does not give much protection. You can also use more starter liquid than the recommended minimum of 10 percent of the total volume of liquid. You can also try to place the kombucha somewhere a bit warmer (78.5 to 80.5 degrees) to speed the fermentation process and makes it go sour faster. To increase the airflow, open the pantry (if that's where the kombucha is) or move the brew to the sink area. Last but not least, it is important that you put the SCOBY in first and then pour the starter liquid on top. By adding a sour starter liquid to the sweet tea, the SCOBY is better protected against mold and other contaminants.

### Soki Choi's tips: Continuous brewing

After you have brewed your first batch of kombucha, you will naturally begin a system of continuous brewing, which means you'll have the opportunity to carry on brewing kombucha on a regular basis. This is how it works: after the first basic brew, you save around 10 percent of the finished basic kombucha (equivalent of around 1¼ cup per 6¼ pints) that can be used as a starter liquid in your next batch.

New potential SCOBY babies are also created after each brew, usually appearing at the top of the kombucha liquid. New SCOBY babies can be used for further brews—or to give away as a gift together with some starter liquid to friends. Older SCOBY (also known as mother SCOBY) can be used as long as they look relatively fresh and no mold has appeared on the surface. A few months up to half a year is not unusual to continue using the mother SCOBY, but to be on the safe side it is always best to brew kombucha using new SCOBYs. Making new kombucha at least once or twice a month is a brewing routine that many try and follow, but find a routine that works for you.

If you get tired of brewing kombucha and want to take a break or go on a holiday, you can pause the process by just letting everything rest. The important thing to keep in mind is that there should be enough liquid in the vessel (at least half) for the SCOBY to float in. The sour environment protects the SCOBY and liquid, which means it is easy to start the brewing again whenever it suits you. Just as when you water plants, the SCOBY likes to be fed with sweet, tepid tea now and again. Store the kombucha in a slightly cooler space if possible (not the fridge). You can press the pause button in this way for a few months. Even if the kombucha gets sourer with time, the liquid can't really get too old as it just turns into healthy kombucha vinegar that can be used in salad dressings and marinades. Of course, I will also share my favorite recipes for kombucha vinegar (p. 167).

CHAPTER 6

# My favorite recipes

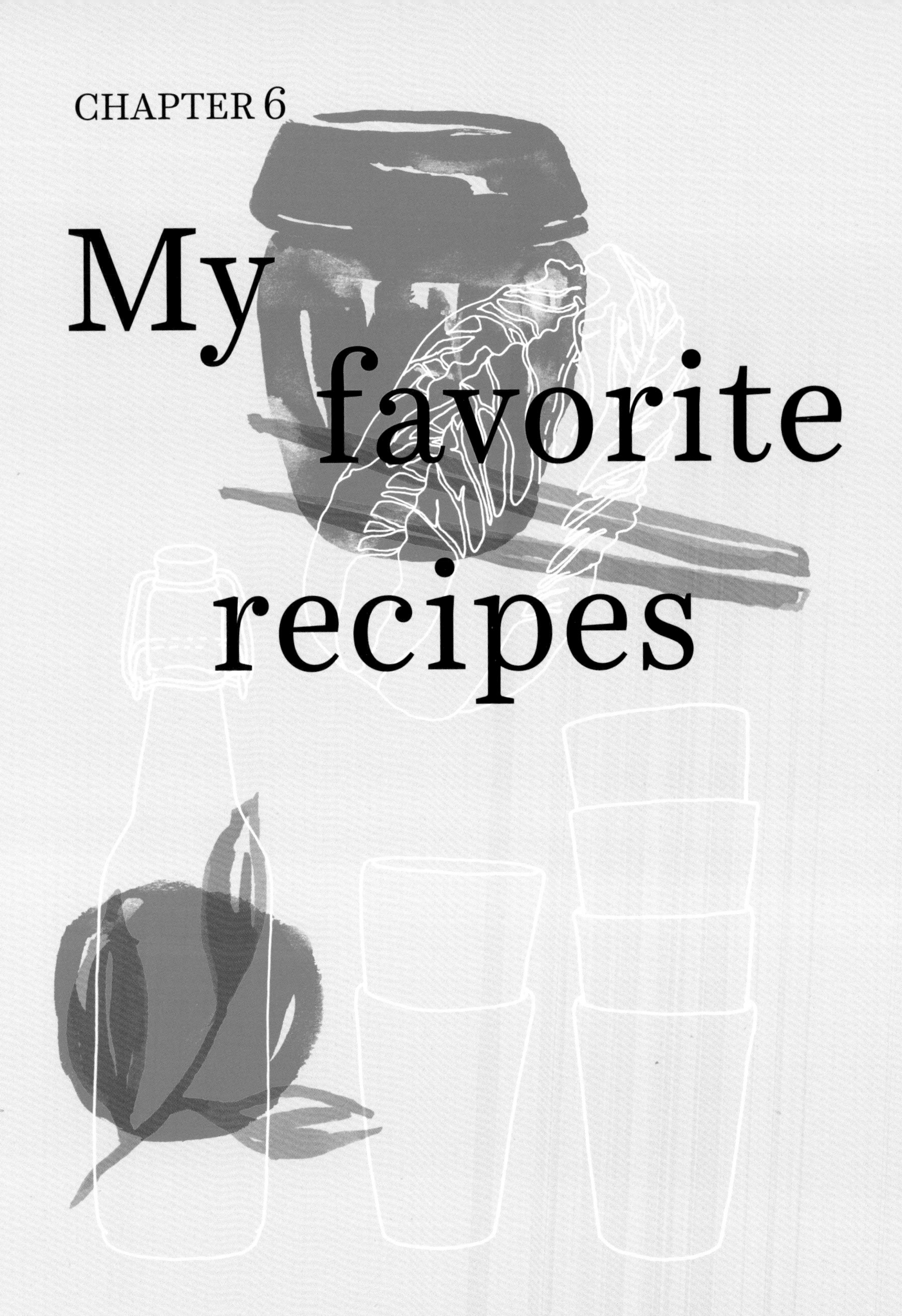

# Kimchi

There is probably no other dish that I have eaten so much of or so passionately as kimchi. According to my mother, kimchi first entered my life when I was around two years old. She carefully dipped bits of kimchi in cold water so that the hot chili and garlic would drip off, and since then kimchi and its bacterial inhabitants have been my constant companions in life. What does kimchi taste like? Heat from chili, saltiness, a refreshing tartness, and seductive umami hits you straight away; I guarantee it tastes like nothing else out there! Just like with other "good/bad" taste experiences (truffle, blue cheeses, and coffee), kimchi can be divisive. Either you fall for it straight away or you don't, so have some patience. Give it time and a couple of chances before you make a definitive decision because, like with all highly complex and deeply flavored foods, you need to get used to it and develop your taste buds.

In this chapter I will share my best recipes for kimchi. You will get my mother's classic kimchi recipe, which, after years of nagging and spying, I managed to get from my mother. Fresh summer kimchi, crunchy cucumber kimchi, and mild white kimchi are other types that will enhance any meal. I'll even share my three favorite signature kimchi dishes. Welcome to my kimchi world!

# Kombucha

My first memory of kombucha was in the 1970s when my father came home with a slimy "mushroom" that he used to make tea. The mushroom was the kombucha culture SCOBY, which was then known as *Volga mushroom*. As usual, I refused to drink any strange health remedy my father experimented with. It wouldn't be until 2013, when I was in Florida, that I would come into contact with my father's fermented tea again. This time it was packed in a nice, colorful bottle and marketed as bubbly probiotic drink, and just like that the bubbly drink slid down my gullet with no problems. When I returned to the United States a few years ago, kombucha was nearly the only thing I would drink, with its complex, tangy, deep taste. For a beginner, it can be difficult to brew kombucha at first, but believe me, it'll become super easy.

To start your brewing, I will share my three best basic recipes for kombucha made with black, white, and green tea. I will also reveal how to make healthy vinegar using "old and sour" kombucha. In addition, I will give you tips on different flavorings that will make your kombucha extra bubbly and tasty. Receiving homebrewed kombucha flavored with mango or blueberry as a gift is something your friends will definitely appreciate—especially because their gut flora and brain will love it!

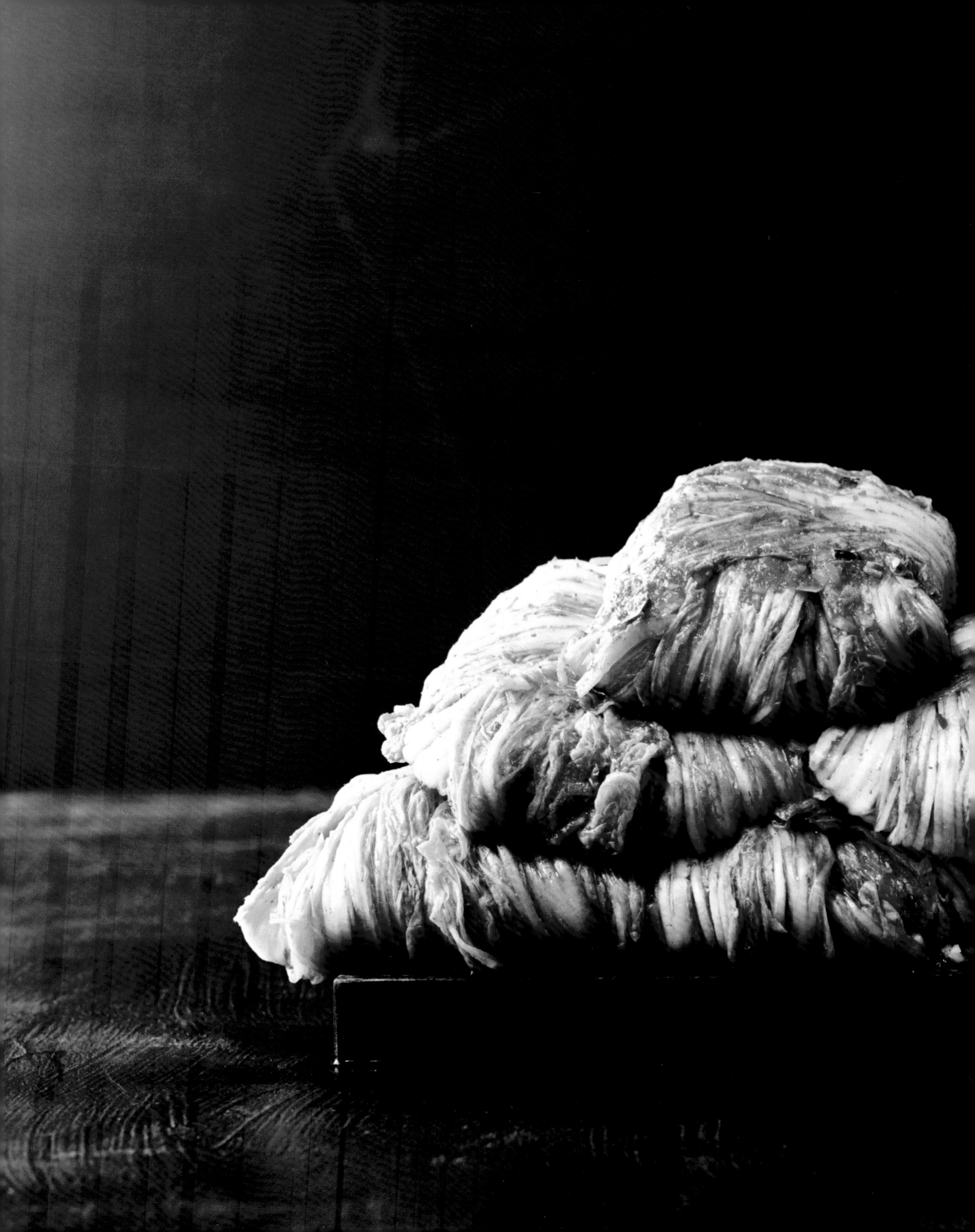

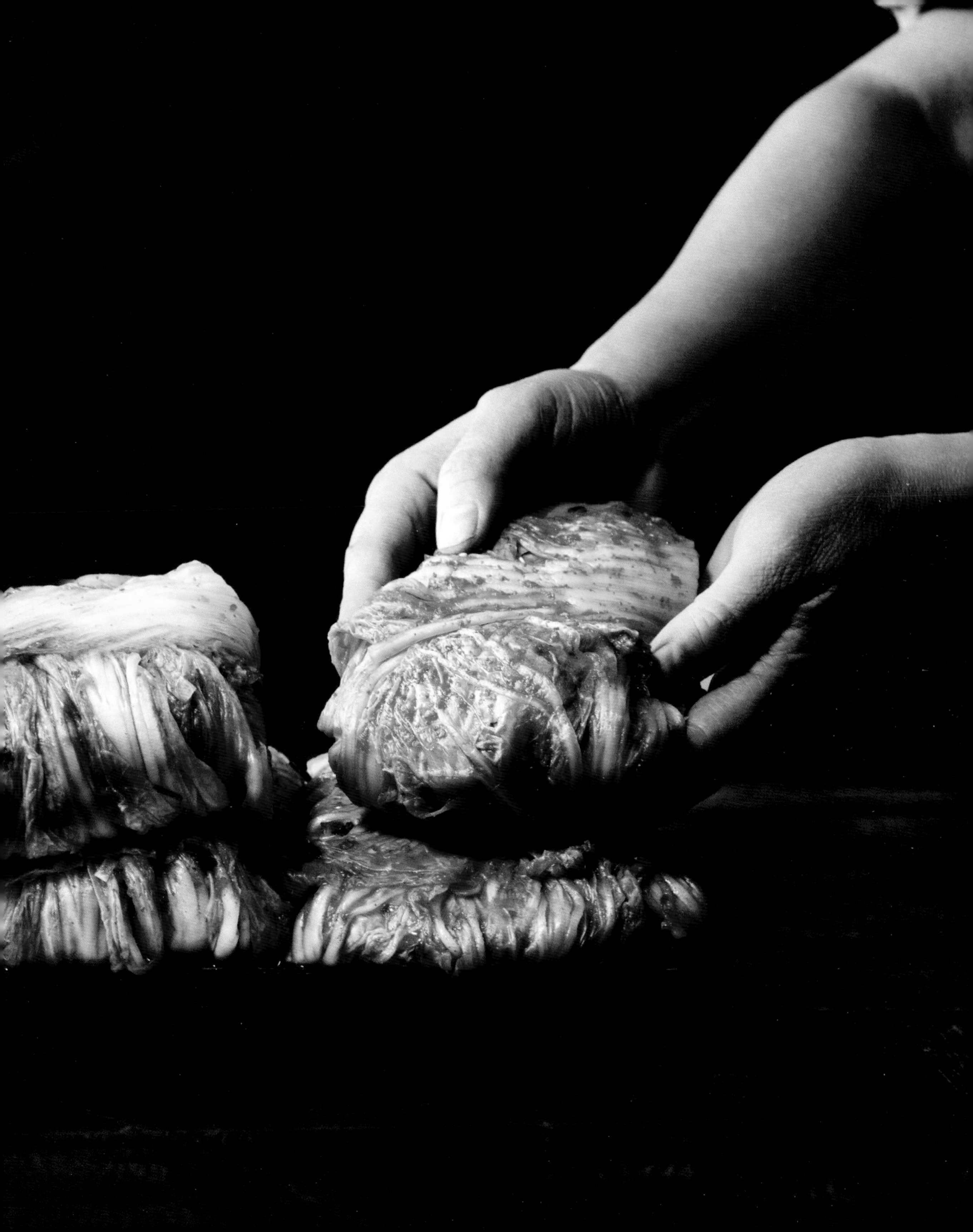

# CLASSIC KIMCHI (my mother's recipe)

This kimchi recipe has been passed down from generation to generation in my mother's family. For a long time, it was a secret only my mother and my aunt knew, but with stubbornness, spying, and a lot of nagging I finally managed to get hold of the recipe that has gotten me and my friends addicted. So here you are. Let me present my mother, Ju, and her recipe for classic kimchi.



**Kimchi base**

Around 3 cabbages (4½ pounds) + couple pinches of salt
10½ pints water + 1 cup salt

**Kimchi mix**

1 teaspoon rice flour + ⅘ cup water
1 small yellow onion, finely chopped
1 apple or pear, grated
1 tablespoon fresh ginger, grated
10 garlic cloves, pressed
2 red chilli peppers, finely chopped
⅖ cup gochugaru
1 ⅗ cups white radish, finely shredded
1 ⅖ cups leek, roughly chopped
1 tablespoon fish sauce
1 tablespoon sugar
1 tablespoon salt

1. Halve the cabbage lengthwise, but not all the way. Take a couple of pinches of salt and salt between each cabbage leaf. See pictures 1–3.
2. Mix 10½ pints of water and 1 cup salt to make a brine and mix until the salt has dissolved. Place cabbage in the brine and place a weight on it so that the cabbage is pressed under the surface. Let it stand for 8 to 9 hours in room temperature (preferably overnight).
3. To make the kimchi mix, boil the rice flour in water while stirring to form a thick paste. Set to one side to cool.
4. Mix the remaining ingredients in a bowl. Add the rice flour mix and stir carefully. Place the kimchi mix and the pickled cabbage in the fridge for 8 hours.
5. Discard the brine from the cabbage and rinse it several times under running water.
6. Place a dollop of kimchi mix in the furthest place in between the leaves near the base and spread the kimchi mix over each leaf. See picture 4.
7. Roll the cabbage halves together (see pictures 5–8) and pack them tightly in a jar with the cut sides facing up. Place a tight-fitting lid on top and let sit at room temperature for 24 hours. Then leave it in the fridge for 4 days to allow the flavor to develop. The longer you leave it, the more tart it becomes. Start to eat once it is sour enough for you.

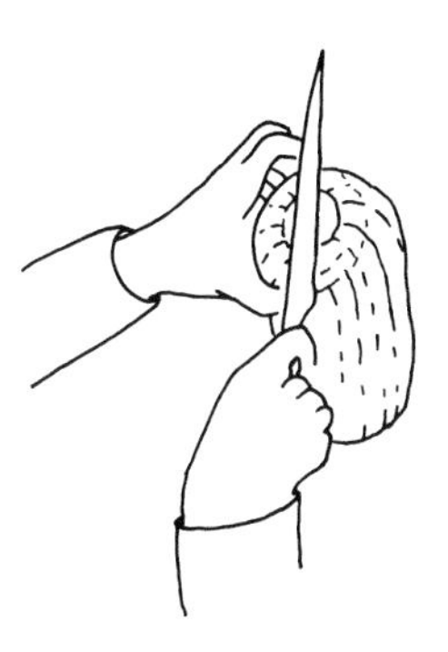

1. Make a 2-inch cut into the root of the cabbage.

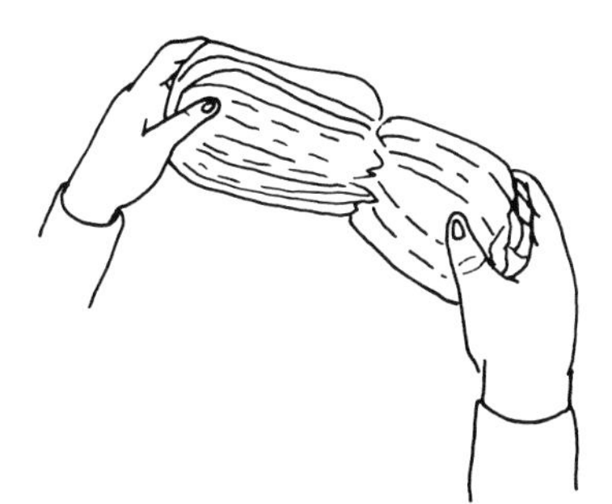

2. Pull the cabbage into two halves but not all the way.

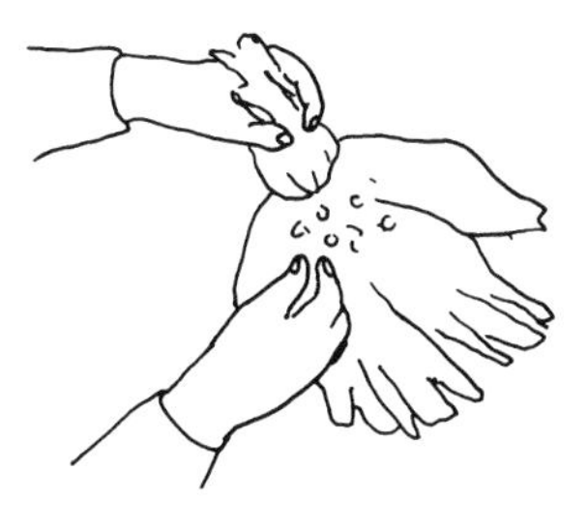

3. Hold the top of the cabbage and spread the bottom leaves outward into a fan shape. Take a couple of pinches of salt and salt between each leaf.

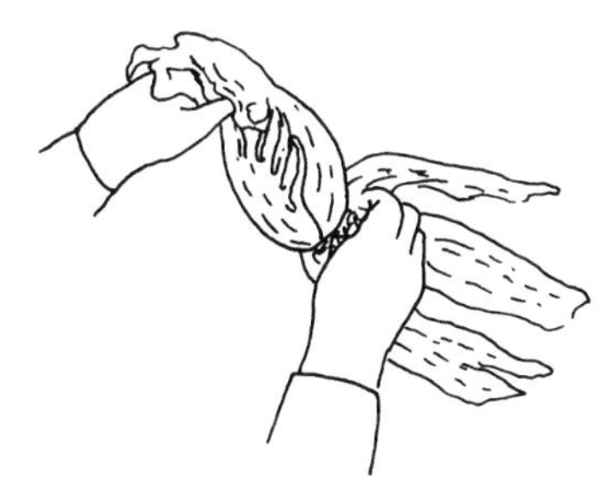

4. Spread out the bottom leaves like a fan. Put a dollop of kimchi mix in the furthest place in between the leaves near the base of the roots and spread the filling out over the leaves. Continue to add kimchi mix on each layer of leaves.

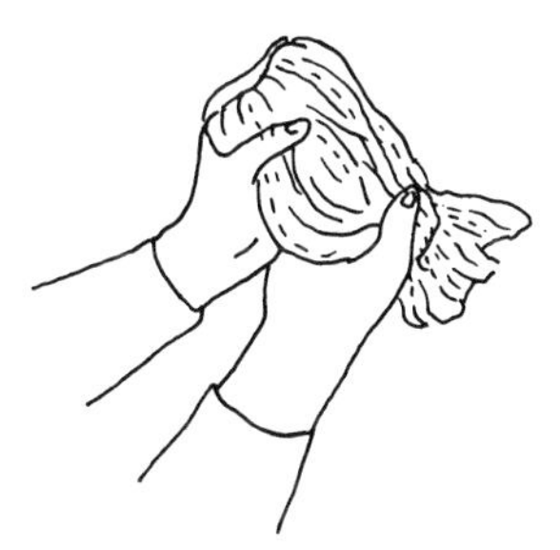

5. Fold the leaves toward the middle of the base so that the cabbage is folded in half.

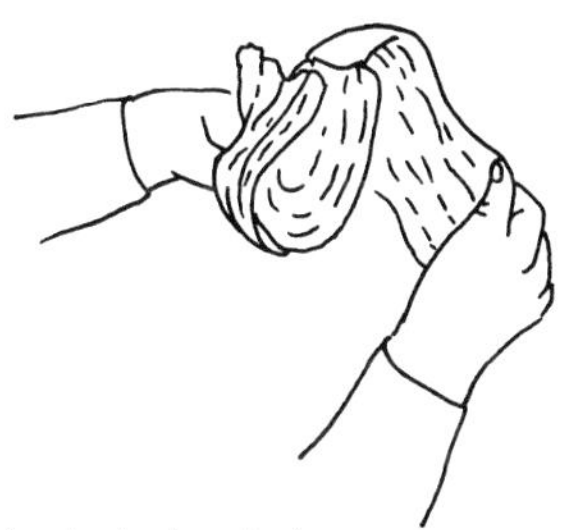

6. Take the leaf at the bottom, pull it slightly to the side, and then smooth over the fold.



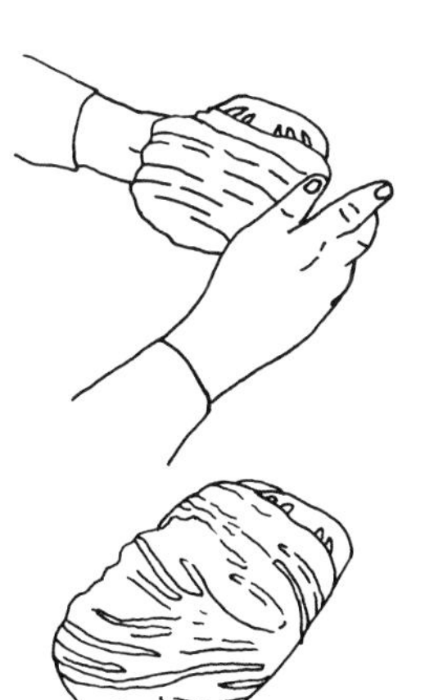

7. Carefully pull the leaf taut over the fold.

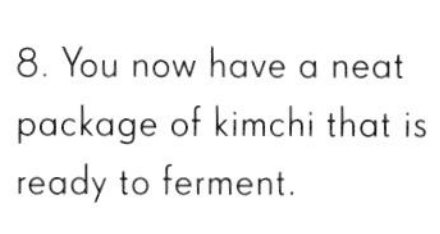

8. You now have a neat package of kimchi that is ready to ferment.

**Gochugaru**

To make authentic kimchi, gochugaru is essential and you can't replace it with, for example, sambal oelek or cayenne pepper. Gochugaru can be found in Asian food stores or larger grocery stores.

**Note!**

Sugar improves the taste of the kimchi and allows for better fermentation. You can remove the sugar if you like, but note that any sugar used will "disappear" during the fermentation process.

## Tips

After four to five days, the kimchi should be ready to eat. It will stay nice and tart for at least a month, then it starts to get sourer and more mature in its taste. Kimchi can never really get too old, so don't throw it out. Really acidic kimchi works perfectly in a kimchi stew (p. 153) and kimchi fried rice (p. 154).

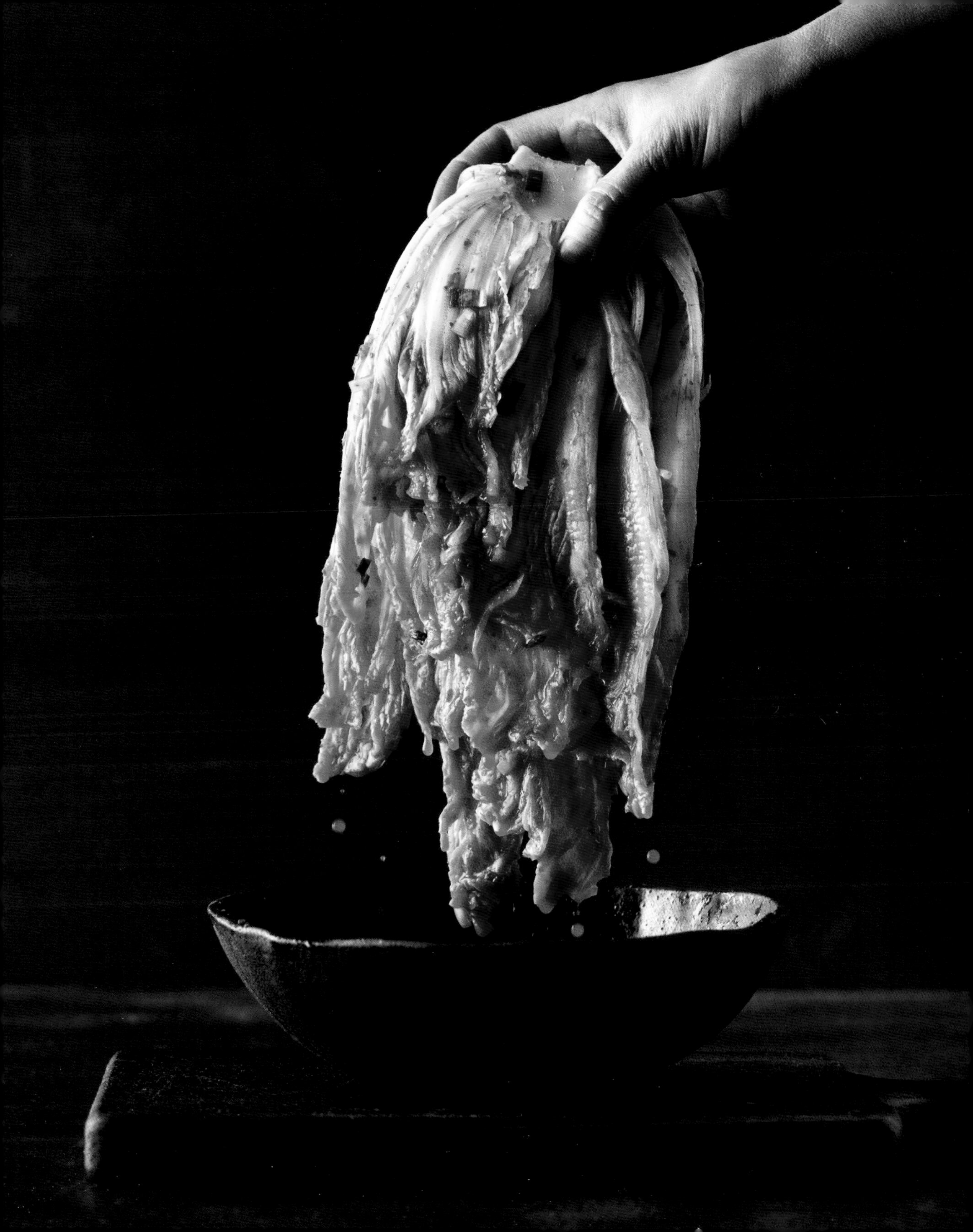

# SOKI'S QUICK KIMCHI

This is my best recipe for quick kimchi that gives the best kimchi in the shortest possible time. If, like me, you are addicted to kimchi, you can always double or quadruple the recipe.

**Kimchi base**

1 cabbage, (1.7–2.2 pounds)
2 tablespoons salt
1 tablespoon water

**Kimchi mix**

½ yellow onion, chopped
¼ apple, roughly chopped
4 garlic cloves, chopped
¾-inch fresh ginger
1 tablespoon water
1 red chili pepper, chopped
1 tablespoon fish sauce
⅖ cup chopped leek
1 teaspoon sugar
1 teaspoon salt
2 tablespoons gochugaru

1. Halve the cabbage lengthwise. Cut the cabbage into bite-size pieces (1 to 1½ inches) and place in a large bowl. Pour in salt and water and mix. Let sit for 2 hours. Mix the cabbage pieces at least once after 1 hour's time.
2. Place the onion, apple, garlic, ginger, water, chili, and fish sauce in a mixer and mix for a short time to make a paste. Add the chopped leek, sugar, salt, and gochugaru, and mix. Set to one side.
3. Rinse the cabbage pieces twice in cold water to remove excess salt. Use a strainer to strain the water. Massage the kimchi mix into the cabbage bits with your hands (you can use plastic gloves).
4. Fill a glass jar with the kimchi cabbage and secure with a tight-fitting lid. Let sit for 24 hours at room temperature. Place in the fridge for at least 4 days.

**Tip!** The fermented fish sauce is important to the fermentation process and gives a deeper umami taste. If you are vegan, replace the fish sauce with one teaspoon of salt.

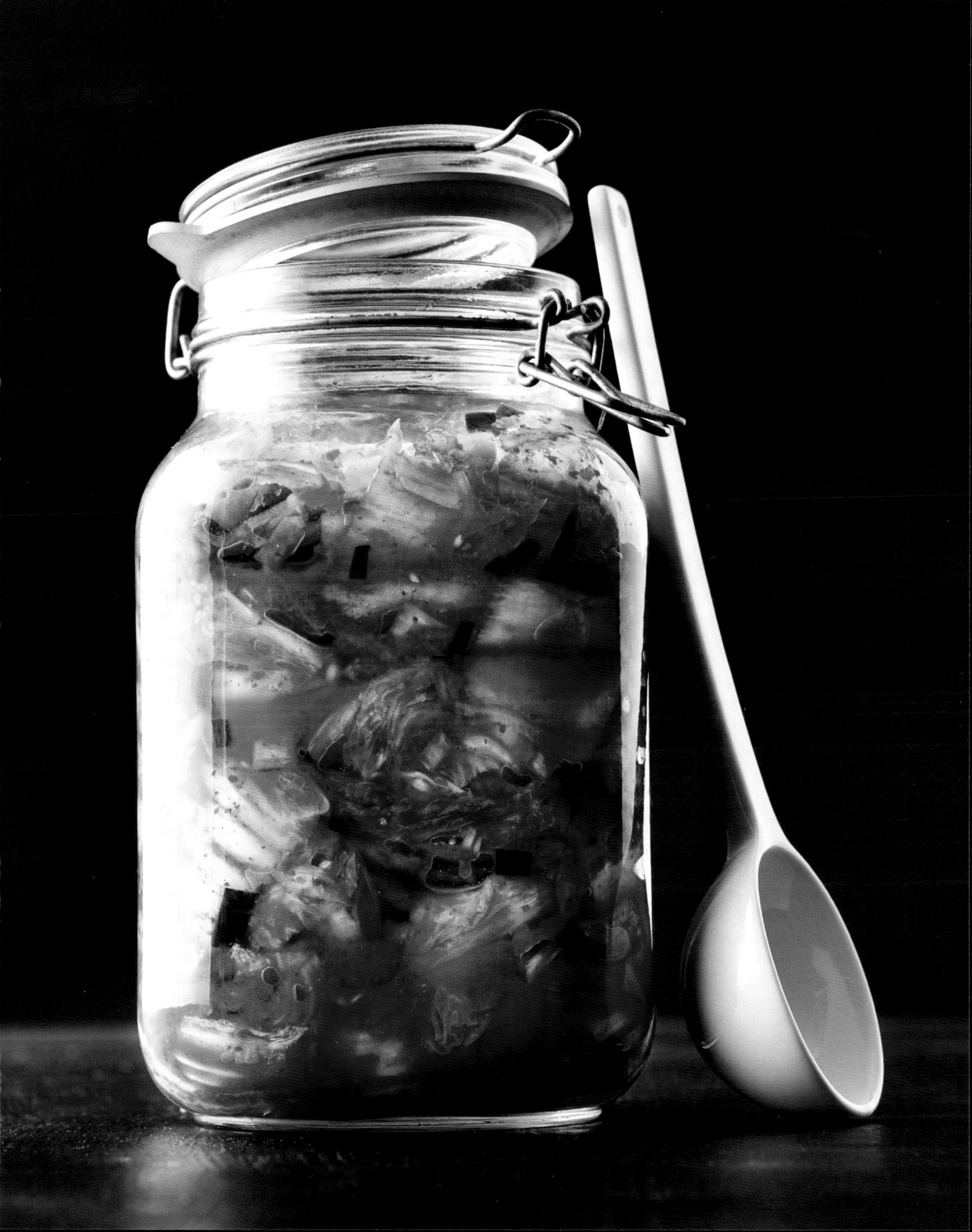

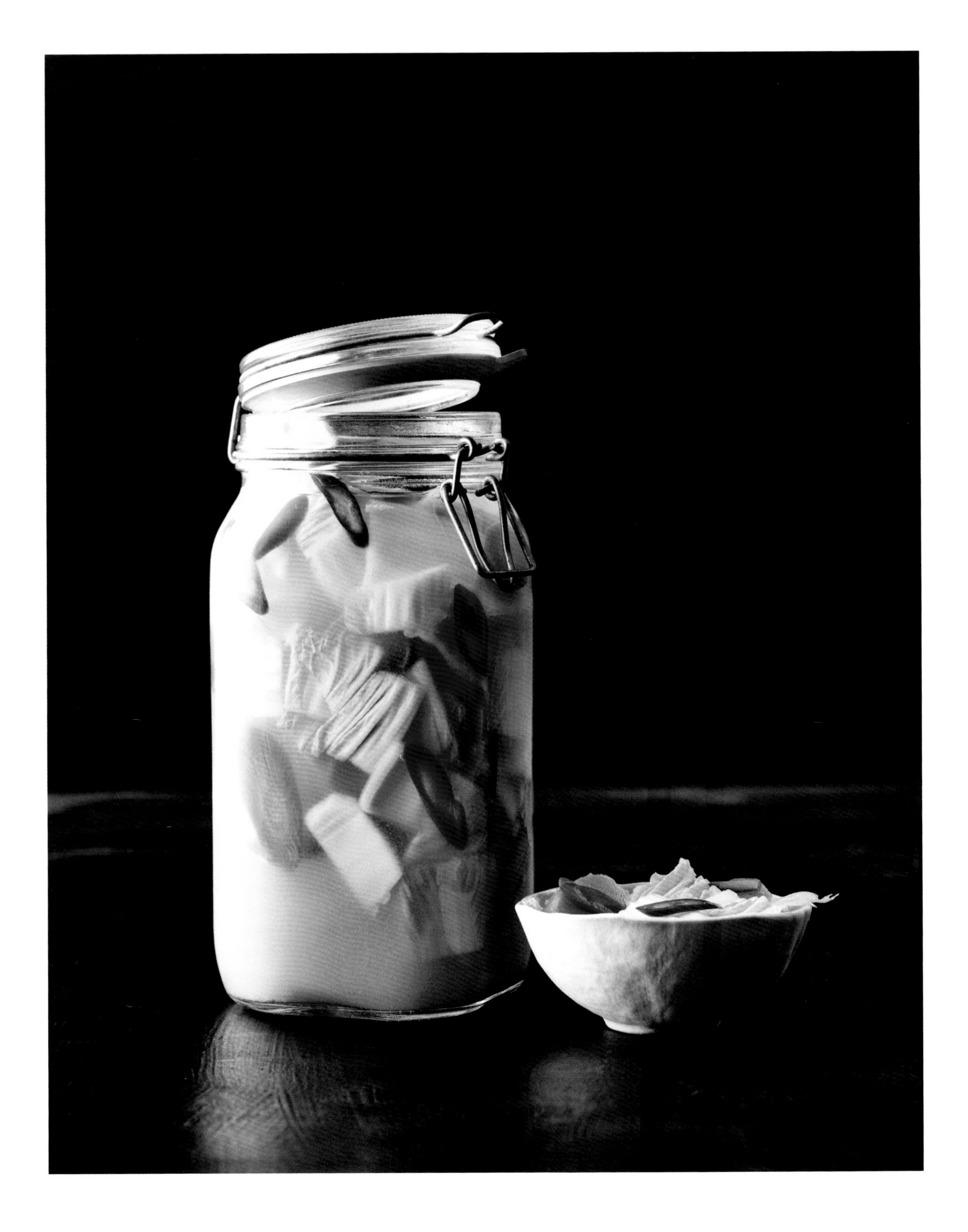

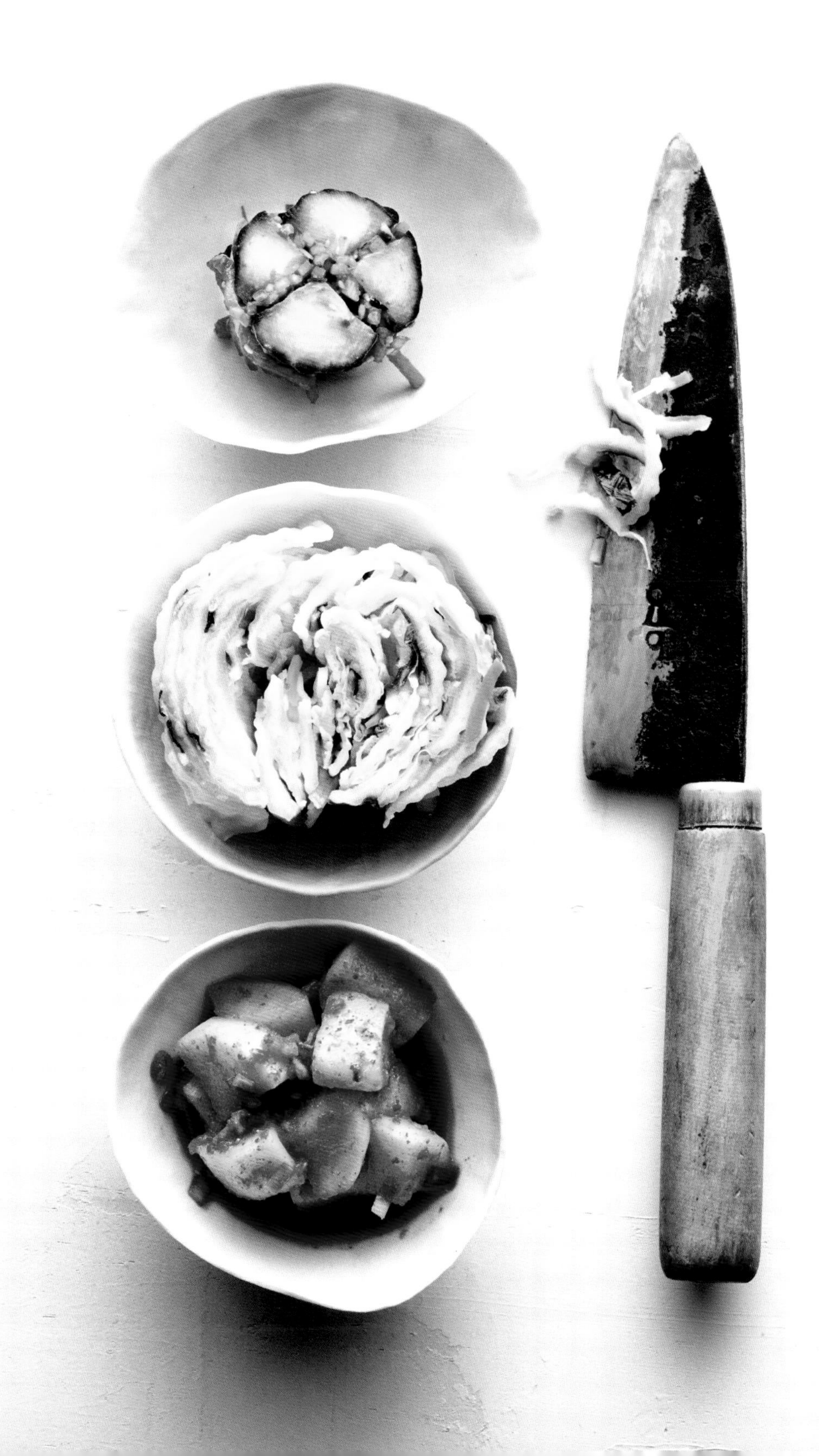

# BAEK KIMCHI: WHITE KIMCHI

White kimchi is a milder version of classic kimchi that gives a nice, fresh taste of apple and ginger (photo on page 147, in the middle).

**Kimchi base**

Around 3 cabbages (around 4½ pounds) + a pinch of salt

10½ pints water + 1 cup salt



**Kimchi mix**

1 tablespoon rice flour + ⅘ cup water

½ apple or pear, finely shredded

5 garlic cloves, finely shredded

1 tablespoon ginger, finely shredded

1¾ cups white radish, finely shredded

2 red chili peppers, thinly sliced

⅘ cup scallions, chopped into ¾-inch pieces

2 teaspoons fish sauce

2 teaspoons sugar

1 tablespoon salt

1. Halve the cabbage lengthwise. Take a pinch of salt and salt each cabbage leaf.
2. Mix water and salt for the brine in a bowl. Mix until the salt has dissolved. Add the cabbage and place a weight on top so it is pressed under the surface. Leave for 8 to 9 hours at room temperature (preferably overnight).
3. Boil rice flour in water while stirring into a thick paste. Take the saucepan off the heat and leave to cool. Mix the remaining ingredients in a bowl. Pour over the rice flour paste and mix carefully.
4. Discard the salt water and rinse the cabbage several times under cold water. Place a dollop of kimchi mix at the base of each leaf and spread the mix over the leaf (use plastic gloves). Make sure the kimchi mix is spread evenly around the cabbage and between the leaves.
5. Roll the cabbage halves together and pack them tightly in a jar with the cut sides facing up. Secure on a tight-fitting lid and let sit at room temperature for 24 hours. Leave in the fridge for at least 4 days. The kimchi will remain tart for 4 to 6 weeks.

# OI KIMCHI: CUCUMBER KIMCHI

Cucumber kimchi has a crispy consistency and is a fresh accompaniment to a barbecue. It is ready to eat after a day or two (photo on page 147, at the top).

**Kimchi base**

3 thin cucumbers (around 2.2 pounds)

3 tablespoons coarse salt

**Kimchi mix**

2 tablespoons gochagaru
2 tablespoons yellow onion, finely chopped
4/5 cup leeks, coarsely chopped
4/5 cup radish, finely shredded
½ tablespoon fish sauce
1 teaspoon fresh ginger, finely grated
1 teaspoon garlic, pressed
½ tablespoon sugar
½ tablespoon salt
1 tablespoon roasted sesame seeds

1. Cut each cucumber into roughly 2-inch-long pieces. Cut a cross in each cucumber piece without cutting through it.
2. Salt the cucumber pieces, stir, and let sit for 30 minutes at room temperature. Stir them again halfway through.
3. Discard the liquid from the cucumber and rinse the cucumber pieces in cold running water. Gently squeeze the liquid from the cucumber.
4. Mix all the ingredients for the kimchi mix in a large bowl. Fill the cuts in the cucumber pieces with the kimchi mix.
5. Place the cucumber kimchi in a glass jar with a tight-fitting lid. Leave in the fridge for at least 1 day. The cucumber kimchi will last around 1 week.

# KAKKDUGI: RADISH KIMCHI

Radish kimchi is a crunchy variety that is slightly sweeter than normal kimchi (photo on page 147, at the bottom).

**Kimchi base**

2 medium-size radishes (around 1.7 pounds)
2 tablespoons coarse salt

**Kimchi mix**

3 tablespoons gochugaru
3 garlic cloves, pressed
½ yellow onion, finely chopped
2 teaspoons fresh ginger, finely grated
½ tablespoon sugar
1 tablespoon fish sauce
4.5 cup leeks, coarsely chopped

1. Peel and cut the radish into ¾-by-¾-inch cubes.
2. Salt the radish, mix, and let sit for 30 minutes at room temperature. Mix them again halfway through.
3. Discard the liquid from the radish, but don't rinse off the salt.
4. Mix all the ingredients for the kimchi mix in a large bowl. Add the radish and mix well.
5. Place the kimchi in a glass jar with a tight-fitting lid. Let sit at room temperature for 24 hours. Then, leave in the fridge for 4 days. The kimchi will last at least 1 month.

# MOL KIMCHI: SUMMER KIMCHI

Summer kimchi is refreshing and thirst-quenching (see photo on p. 146).

**Kimchi mix**

1 tablespoon rice flour + 3 cups water
1 teaspoon fish sauce
½ tablespoon salt
½ tablespoon sugar

**Vegetables**

½ cabbage (around 0.8 pounds), chopped into ¾-inch pieces
⅖ cup scallions, chopped into ¾-inch pieces
1 garlic clove, thinly sliced
1 teaspoon finely shredded ginger
½ carrot, thinly sliced (slanted)
½ apple, chopped into 1-inch sticks
1 red chili pepper, thinly sliced

1. Mix rice flour and water in a saucepan and bring to a boil while stirring. Remove the saucepan from the heat and leave it to cool.
2. Add the fish sauce, salt, and sugar to the rice flour mix and stir. Put to the side.
3. Put all the cut vegetables and apple in a large glass jar with a tight-fitting lid. Stir the vegetables to distribute them evenly.
4. Pour the kimchi mix over the vegetables. Let sit at room temperature for 24 hours. Place the kimchi in the fridge for at least 2 days. Summer kimchi will keep tart for 2 to 3 weeks.



# SALMON WITH KIMCHI

Kimchi doesn't always have to be a side dish; it also a good ingredient in larger meals. Salmon with kimchi is one of my lunch favorites, and it can be quickly thrown together.

2 servings

0.2 pounds (100 grams) salmon
Some iceberg lettuce
1¾ cups short-grain rice, cooked
1 avocado, diced
⅘ cup kimchi slices
2 teaspoons sesame oil
2 tablespoons roasted nori (seaweed)
2 teaspoons roasted sesame seeds

**Gochujang sauce**

2 tablespoons gochujang
1 tablespoon honey
3 teaspoons rice vinegar

1. Slice the salmon into ¼-inch slices.
2. Add some iceberg lettuce to the bottom of two deep plates. Add rice, avocado, kimchi, and the sliced salmon. Splash with some sesame oil and garnish with nori and sesame seeds.
3. Mix the ingredients for the gochujang sauce in a bowl.
4. Add the gochujang sauce over the food, mix, and enjoy!

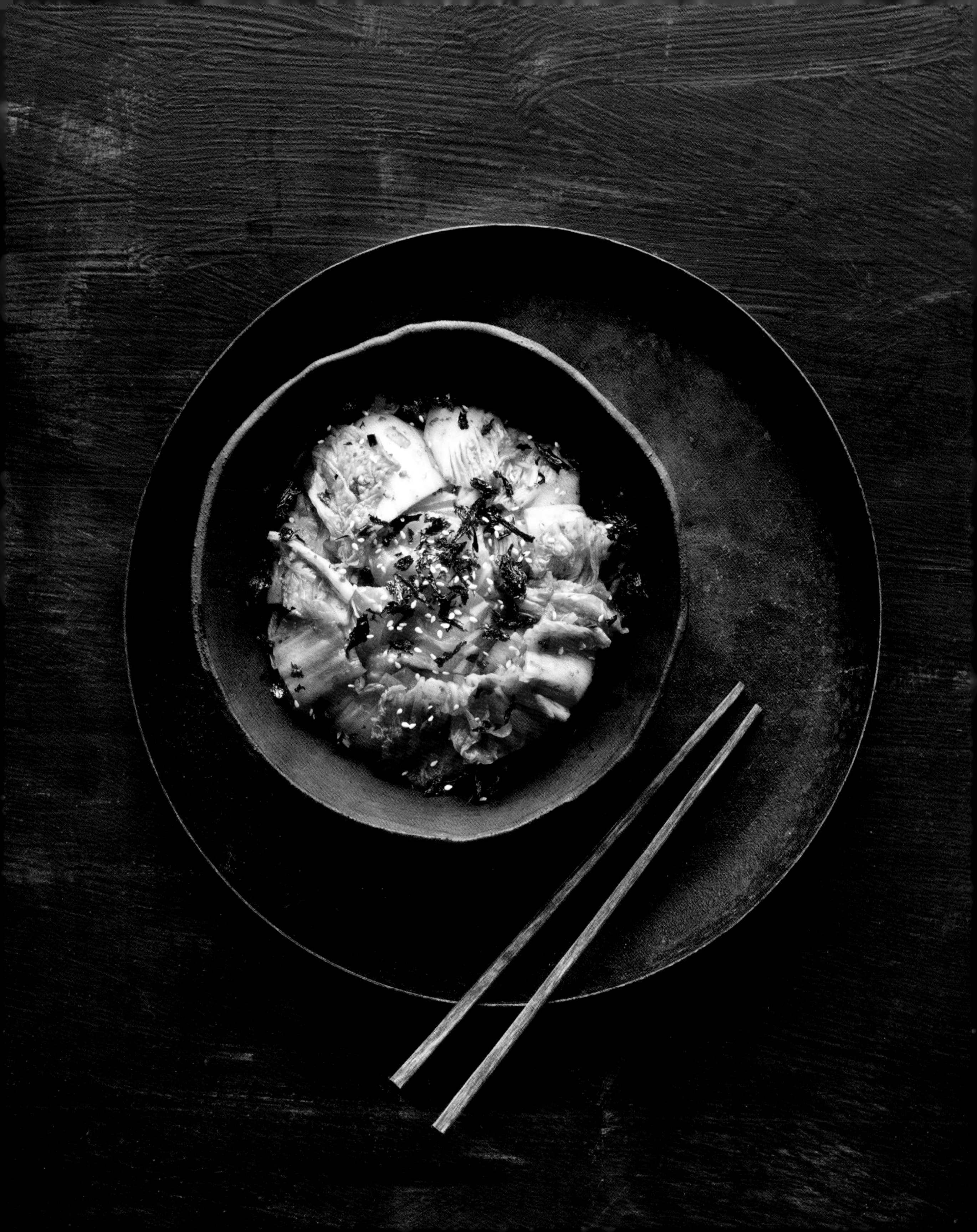

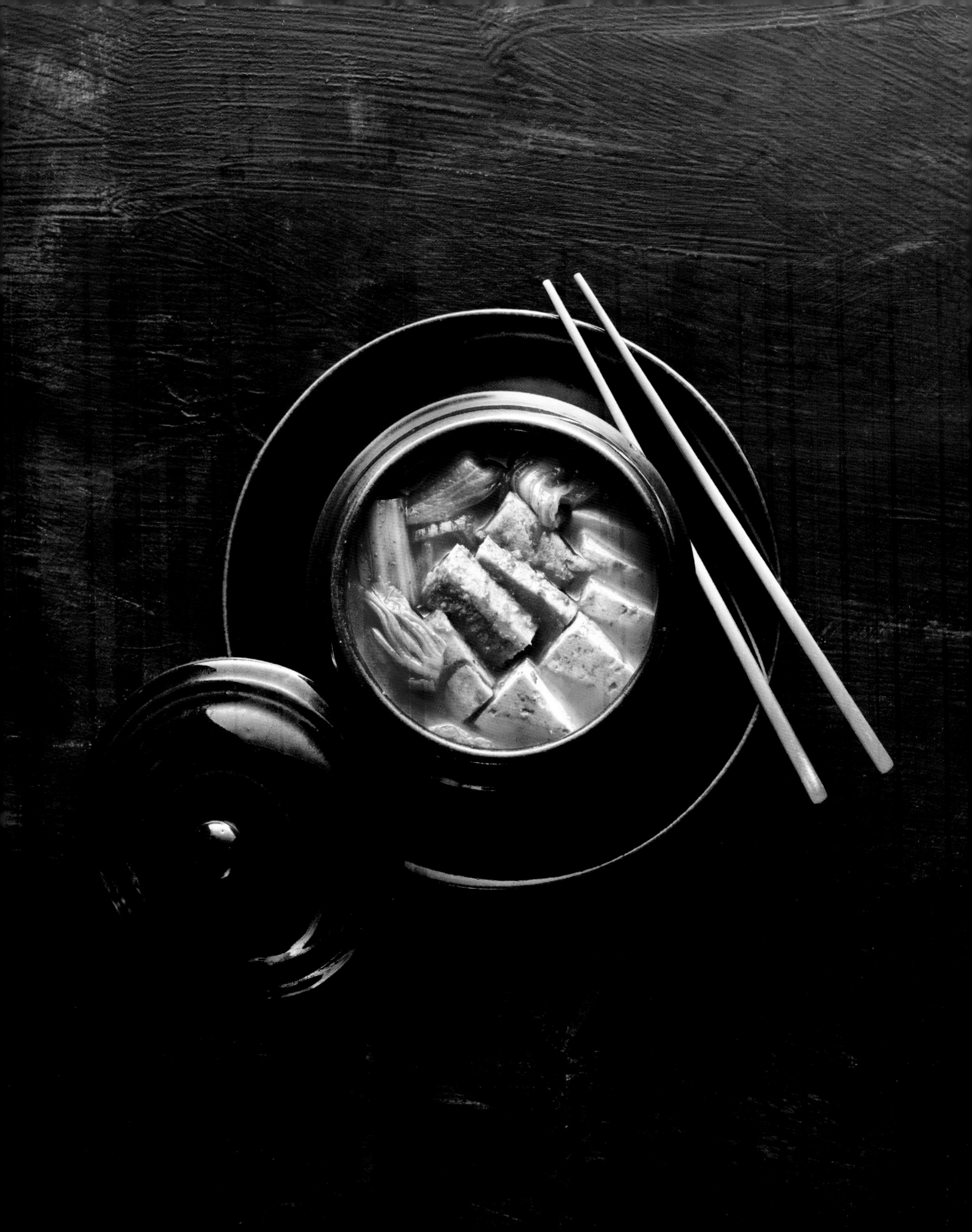

# KIMCHI JJIGAE: KIMCHI STEW

This is a classic in Korea and my favorite dish of all. Musty, hot, and filling, it's made from really mature and tangy kimchi. Try it!

2–3 servings

- 1 tablespoon canola oil or sunflower oil
- 0.8 pounds (400 grams) tart kimchi
- ½ yellow onion, coarsely chopped
- 1 garlic clove, pressed
- 1¾ cups water
- ½ fish stock cube
- 1 can tuna fish in oil
- 1 teaspoon gochugaru
- 0.4 pounds (200 grams) firm tofu
- ⅖ cup leeks, coarsely chopped
- Black pepper
- Cooked rice to serve

1. Heat the oil in a pot and fry kimchi, yellow onion, and garlic over high heat.
2. Add water so the kimchi and onion are covered. Add the fish stock cube, tuna, and gochugaru. Lid and simmer on medium heat for 10 minutes.
3. Add large pieces of tofu and leek. Add black pepper to taste. Stir and simmer for 5 more minutes.
4. Serve with cooked rice.

Tip!

Don't throw any leftover rice away. Cold rice acts as a prebiotic boost for your brain. Read more on page 93.

# KIMCHI BOK KUM BAP: KIMCHI FRIED RICE

This dish is perfect for when you have cold, cooked leftover rice in the fridge from last night's dinner. Combined with kimchi and vegetables, you can make a great dinner in next to no time with lots of resistant starch.

2–3 servings

½ yellow onion, roughly chopped
½ carrot, diced
½ red pepper, diced
6–8 sliced mushrooms
1 tablespoon canola oil or sunflower oil
1 tablespoon light soy sauce
Freshly ground black pepper
0.4 pounds (200 grams) tart kimchi
0.8 pounds (400 grams) cold, cooked rice
⅖ cup frozen peas
1 tablespoon gochujang
1 teaspoon sesame oil
Sesame seeds to garnish
Sliced scallions to garnish
Lime to serve

1. Fry onion, carrot, pepper, and mushrooms in some oil in a pot over high heat until they start to color and soften. Season with soy sauce and a few grinds of pepper.
2. Squeeze all the liquid from the kimchi and shred it into ½-inch pieces.
3. Add kimchi, cold rice, and peas. Fry for another 5 minutes. Mix in the gochujang and sesame oil, and fry for another minute or so.
4. Garnish with sesame seeds, scallions, and lime. Serve immediately.

Tip!
Gochujang is a fermented umami chili paste from Korea that you can find in larger grocery stores.

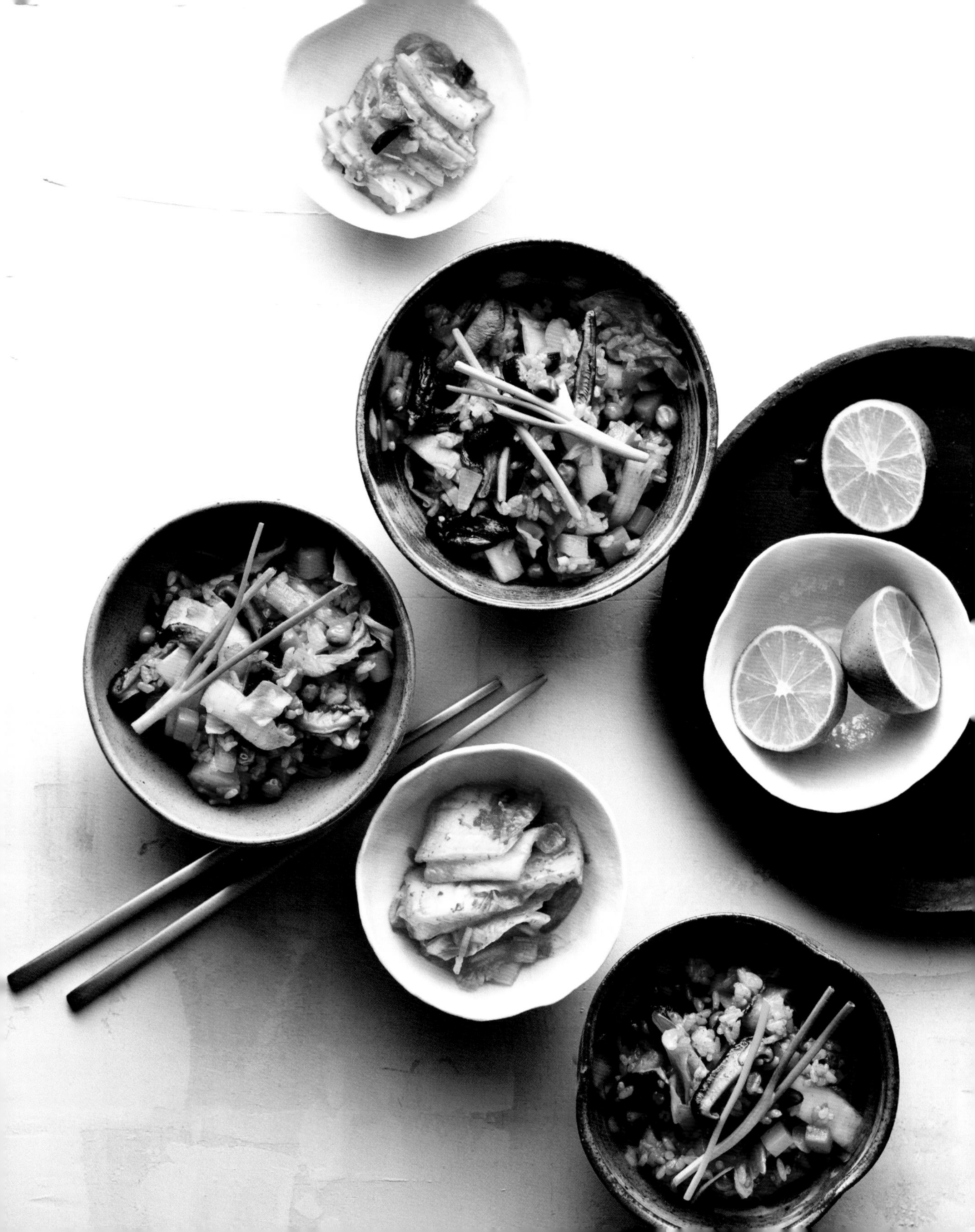

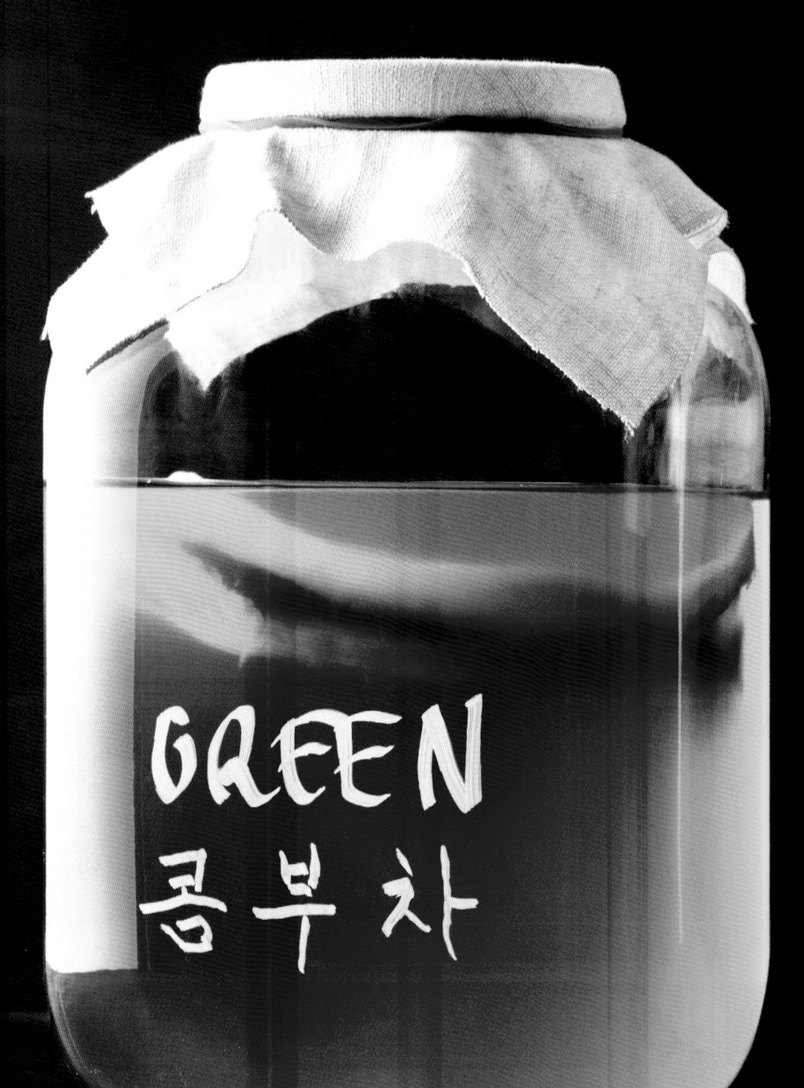
GREEN
콤부차

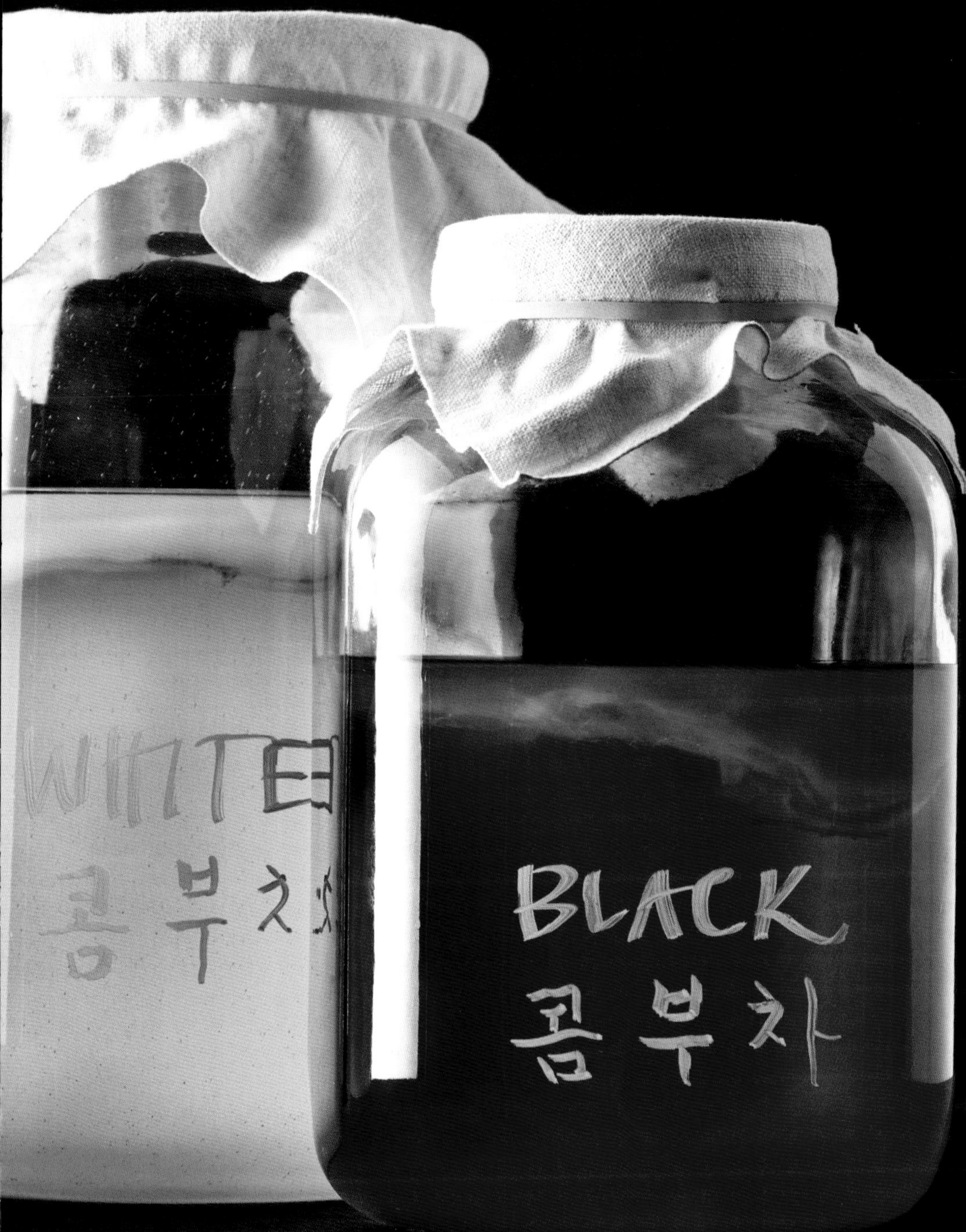
BLACK
콤부차

# Basic Kombucha brew—three types

Kombucha can either be natural or flavored. Start by finding your favorite natural kombucha and then experiment with different flavorings. Read more about where to find SCOBY on page 126.

## BLACK: KOMBUCHA FROM BLACK TEA

6.3 pints

- 5 pints water
- 3 tablespoons black tea (or 6 tea bags)
- 1¼ cups raw sugar
- 2½ cups kombucha (starter liquid)
- 1 SCOBY

1. Boil the water. Add the tea, pour in the sugar, and stir. Let it cool to room temperature (around 77°F).
2. Sieve to remove the tea leaves or remove the tea bags. Pour the liquid into a clean glass container.
3. Add kombucha (starter liquid) and then the SCOBY. Use a cotton cloth as a lid and secure on top of the container, making sure it is taut. Let sit at room temperature for 7 to 12 days untouched.
4. Do a taste test starting from day 7 with a straw until it tastes the way you want it. Place it in the fridge where it will keep for several months. The longer it stands, the more tart it will become.

## WHITE: KOMBUCHA FROM WHITE TEA

8½ pints

- 6¼ pints water
- 4 tablespoons white tea (or 8 tea bags)
- 1¼ cups raw sugar
- 2 pints kombucha (starter liquid)
- 1 SCOBY

1. Bring the water to a boil, add the tea, pour in the sugar, and stir. Let it cool down to room temperature (around 77°F).
2. Sieve to remove the tea leaves or remove the tea bags. Pour into a clean glass container.
3. Add the kombucha (starter liquid) and add the SCOBY. Use a cotton cloth as a lid and secure on top of the container, making sure it is taut. Leave at room temperature for 7 to 12 days untouched.
4. Do a taste test starting from day 7 with a straw until it tastes the way you want it. Place it in the fridge where it will keep several months. The longer it stands, the more tart it will become.

## GREEN: FAST KOMBUCHA WITH GREEN TEA

6¼ cups

- 2 + 3¾ pints cold water
- 3 tablespoons green tea (or 6 tea bags)
- 3/5 cup raw sugar
- 4/5 cup kombucha (starter liquid)
- 1 SCOBY

1. Boil 2 pints of water. Add the tea, add sugar, and stir. Leave to steep for 10 minutes.
2. Sieve to remove the tea or remove the tea bags. Pour in the remaining 3¾ pints of water. Pour into a clean glass jar.
3. Add the kombucha (starter liquid) and add the SCOBY. Use a cotton cloth as a lid and secure on top of the container, making sure it is taut. Leave at room temperature for 7 to 12 days untouched.
4. Do a taste test starting from day 7 with a straw until it tastes the way you want it. Place it in the fridge, where it will keep for several months. The longer it stands, the more tart it will become.

**Sugar!**
Remember that sugar is needed to feed the kombucha culture, otherwise it will die. The sugar converts to organic acids and other healthy substances over time.

## FLAVORED KOMBUCHA

You can flavor your kombucha after you have made the basic brew with freshly pressed juice of your choice (1 part juice + 4 parts kombucha) or fruit and berries (1 part fruit and berries + 4 parts kombucha). It is important that the juice does not contain any preservatives or additives. Before you flavor your kombucha, make sure you remove around 10 percent (1¼ to 1¾ cups) of the unflavored kombucha and keep it in a clean glass jar using a tightly secured piece of cloth as a lid. This will be your starter liquid for the next time you make kombucha.

**Instructions:** Add your preferred flavor to clean bottles first and then fill with kombucha all the way to the top. Leave the bottles, well-sealed, at room temperature for 2 to 4 days to allow it to naturally build up carbonation (post-fermentation). Finally, place the bottles in the fridge and enjoy; it will keep at least a month.

## MY FAVORITE FLAVORS

- Blueberry
- Mango
- Strawberry and rhubarb
- Apple and mint
- Pear and ginger
- Cucumber and mint

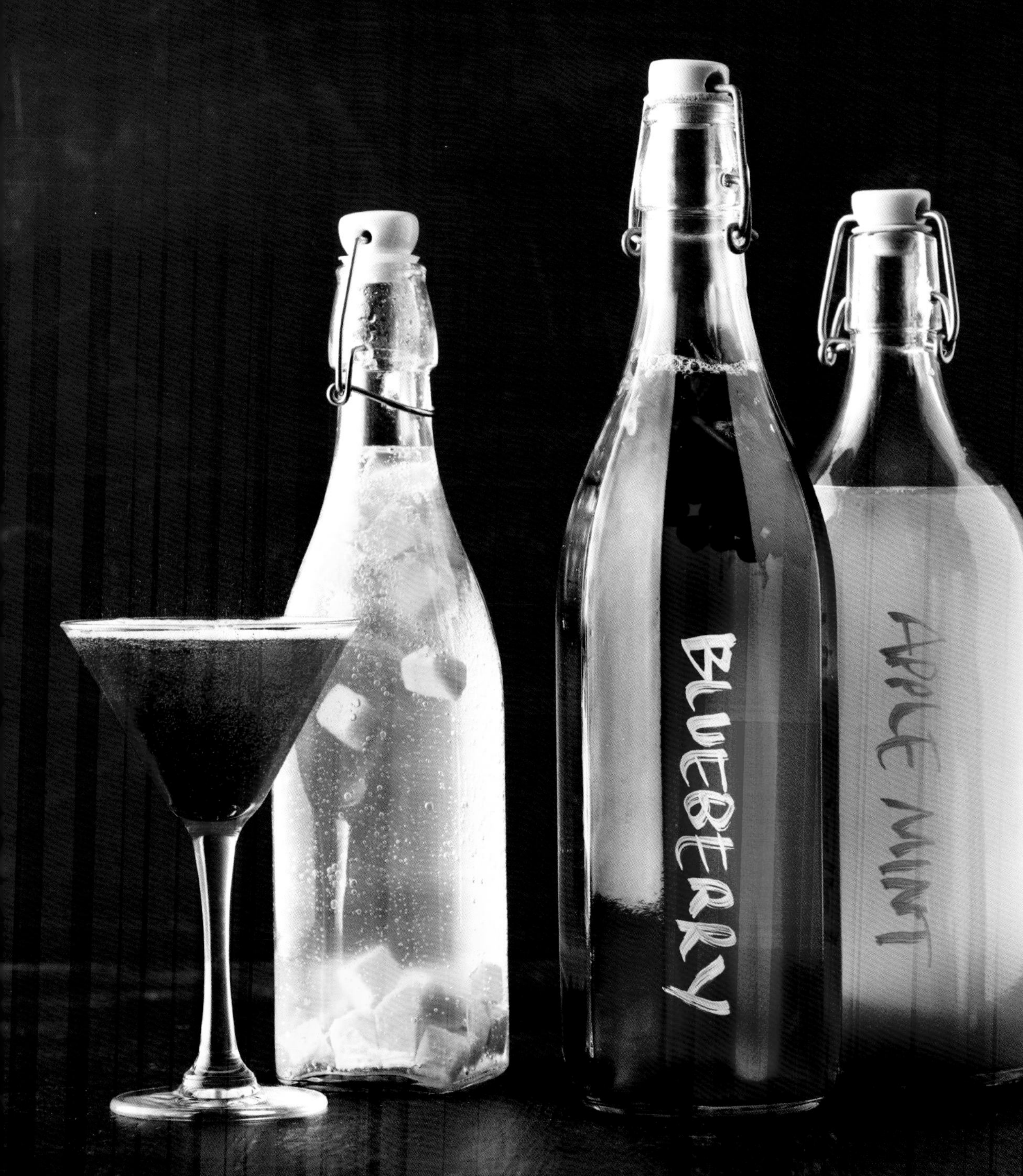
BLUEBERRY
APPLE MINT

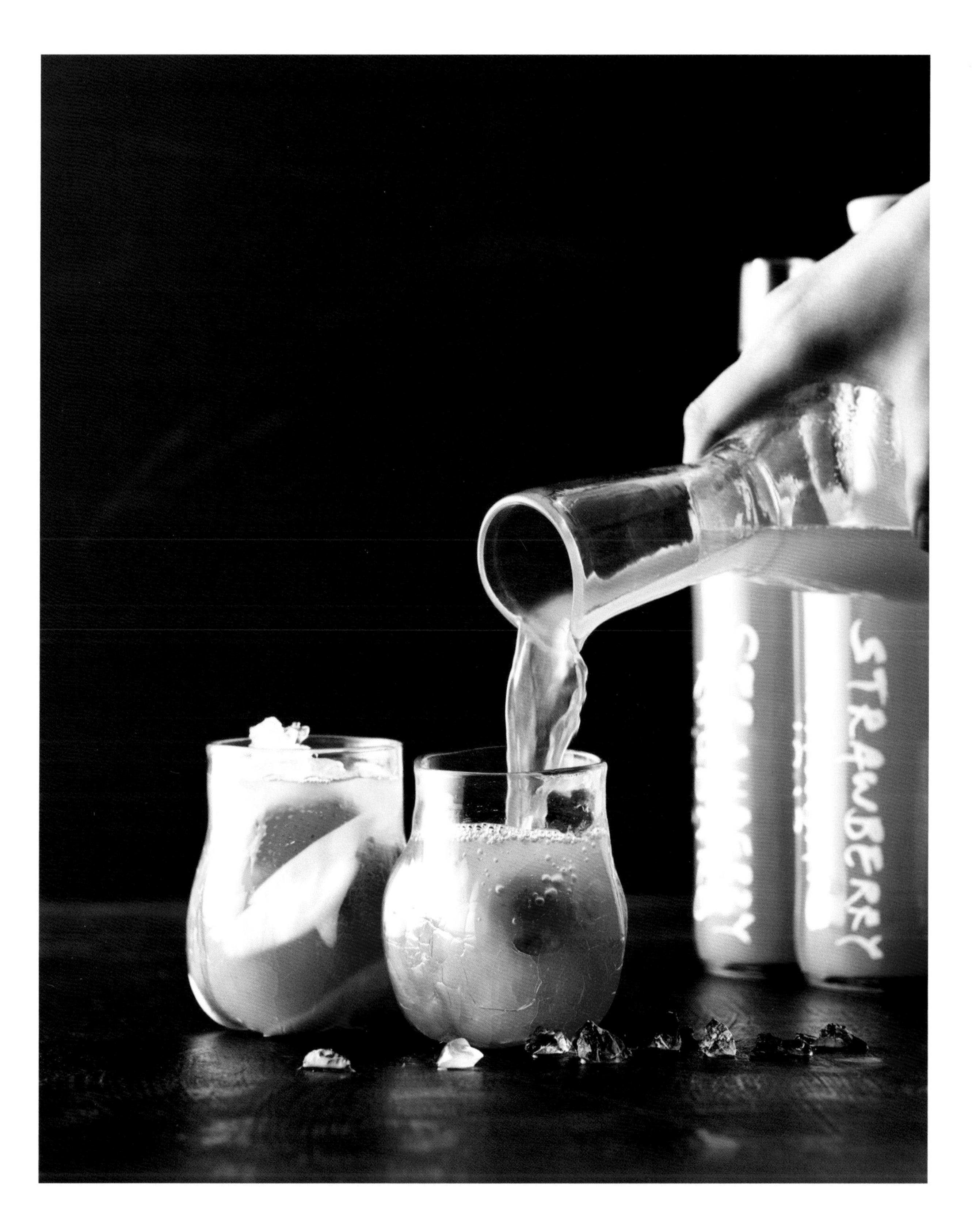
STRAWBERRY

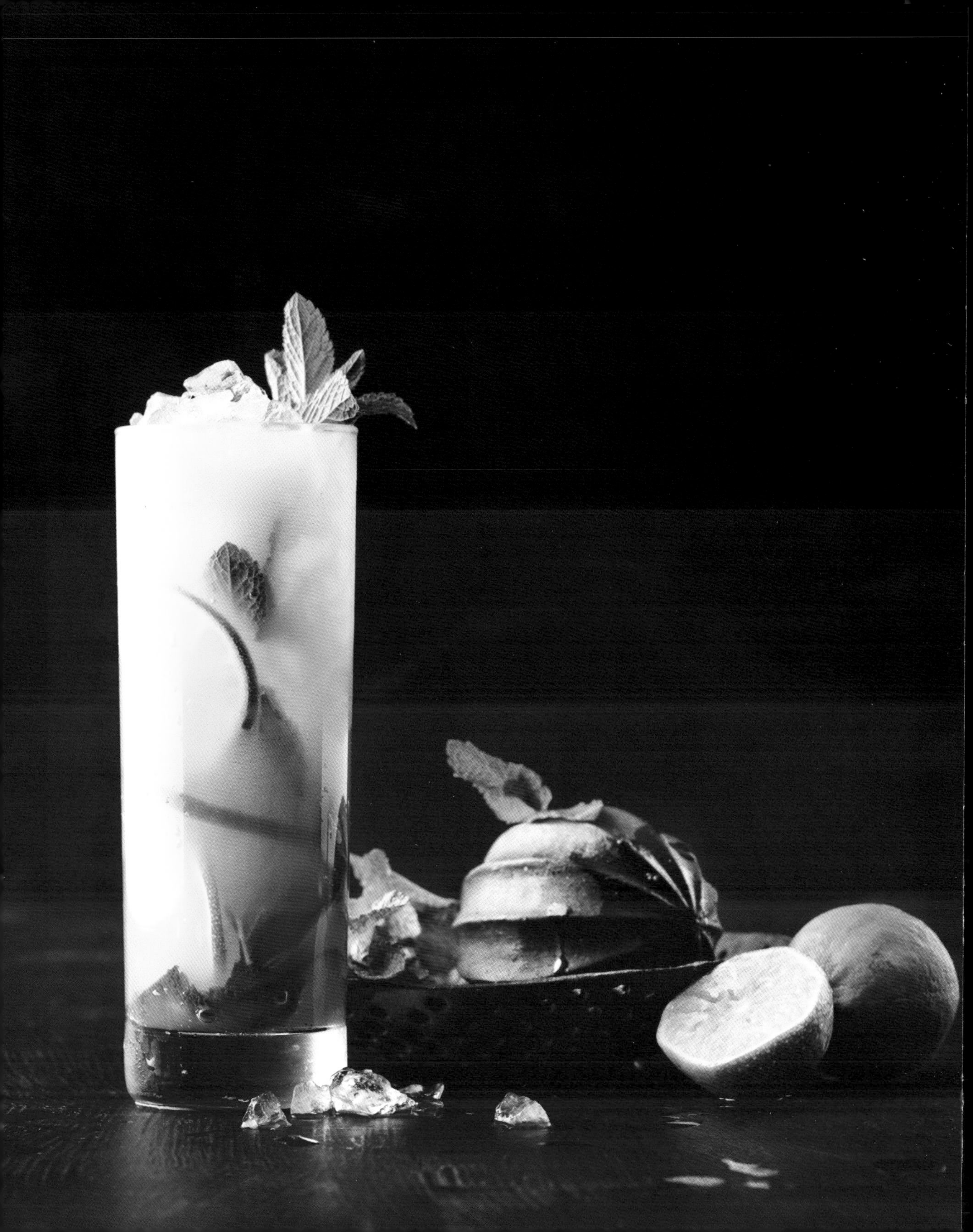

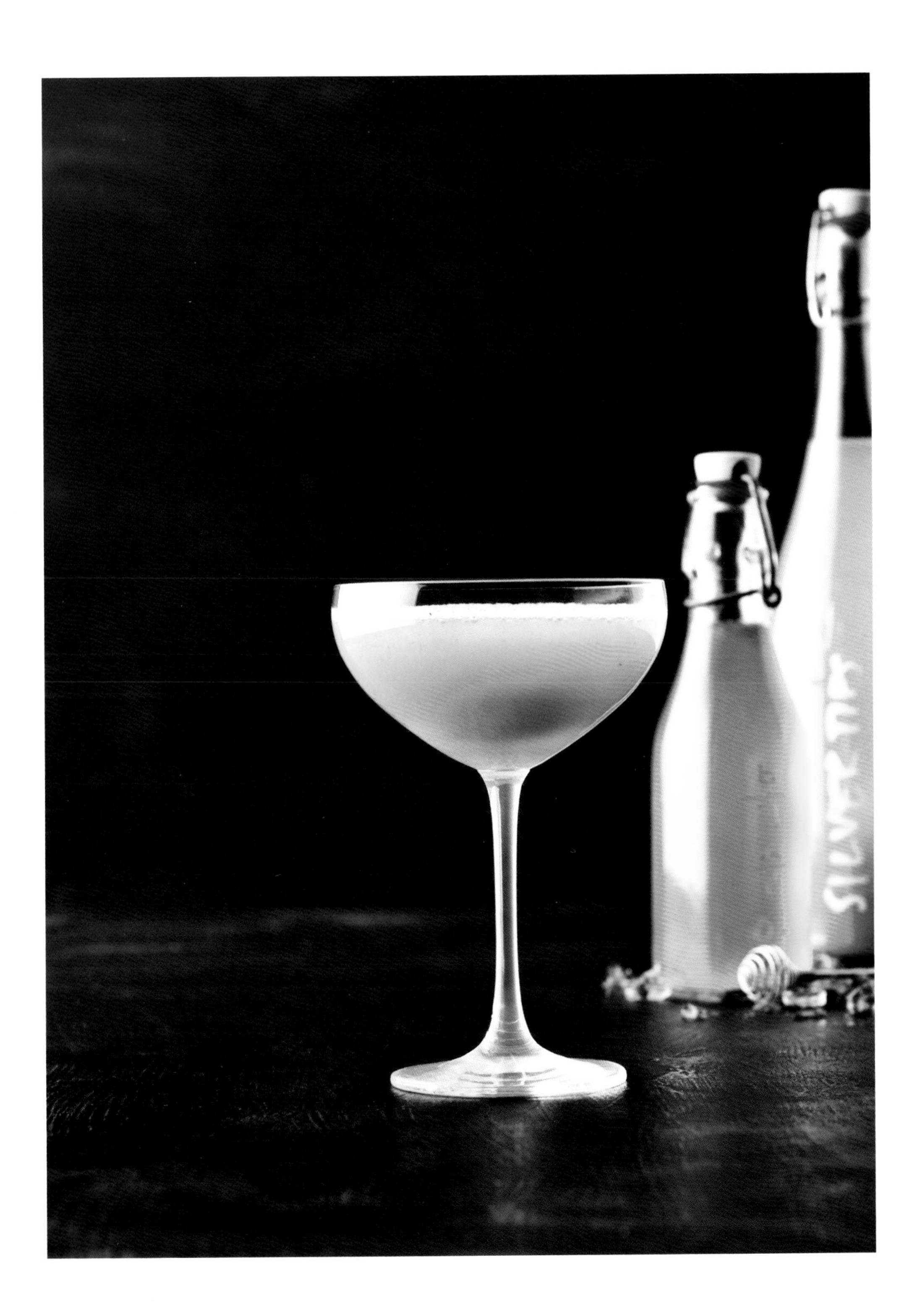

# Kombucha cocktails

Besides tasting good and being healthy, kombucha is also a wonderful alternative to beer and wine, and, above all, a great base for good drinks! These are my favorite recipes.

## KOMBUCHA MOJITO

1 glass

- 10 fresh mint leaves
- ½ lime, cut in 4 segments
- 1 tablespoon raw sugar
- Crushed ice
- ⅖ cup cold kombucha (preferably flavored with apple and mint)
- Club soda
- 1 sprig of mint

**Instructions:** Muddle mint leaves, lime segments, and sugar in a tall glass. Fill with crushed ice and kombucha, preferably flavored with apple and mint. Top off with club soda. Garnish with a sprig of mint and serve immediately.



## KOMBUCHA BELLINI

3 glasses

- 4 tablespoons white peach puree
- ⅖ cup cold kombucha (preferably white, see p. 158)
- ⅖ cup club soda

**Instructions:** Separate the peach puree into three champagne glasses. Fill with kombucha and stir. Top with club soda and serve immediately.

## KOMBUCHA COSMO

2 glasses

- ⅖ cup cranberry juice
- ⅖ cup cold kombucha
- 1½ tablespoons lime juice (juice from around 2 limes)
- Ice
- Shredded lime peel to garnish

**Instructions:** Shake the cranberry juice, kombucha, and lime juice properly in a shaker with ice. Pour into chilled cocktail glasses. Garnish with lime peel and serve immediately.

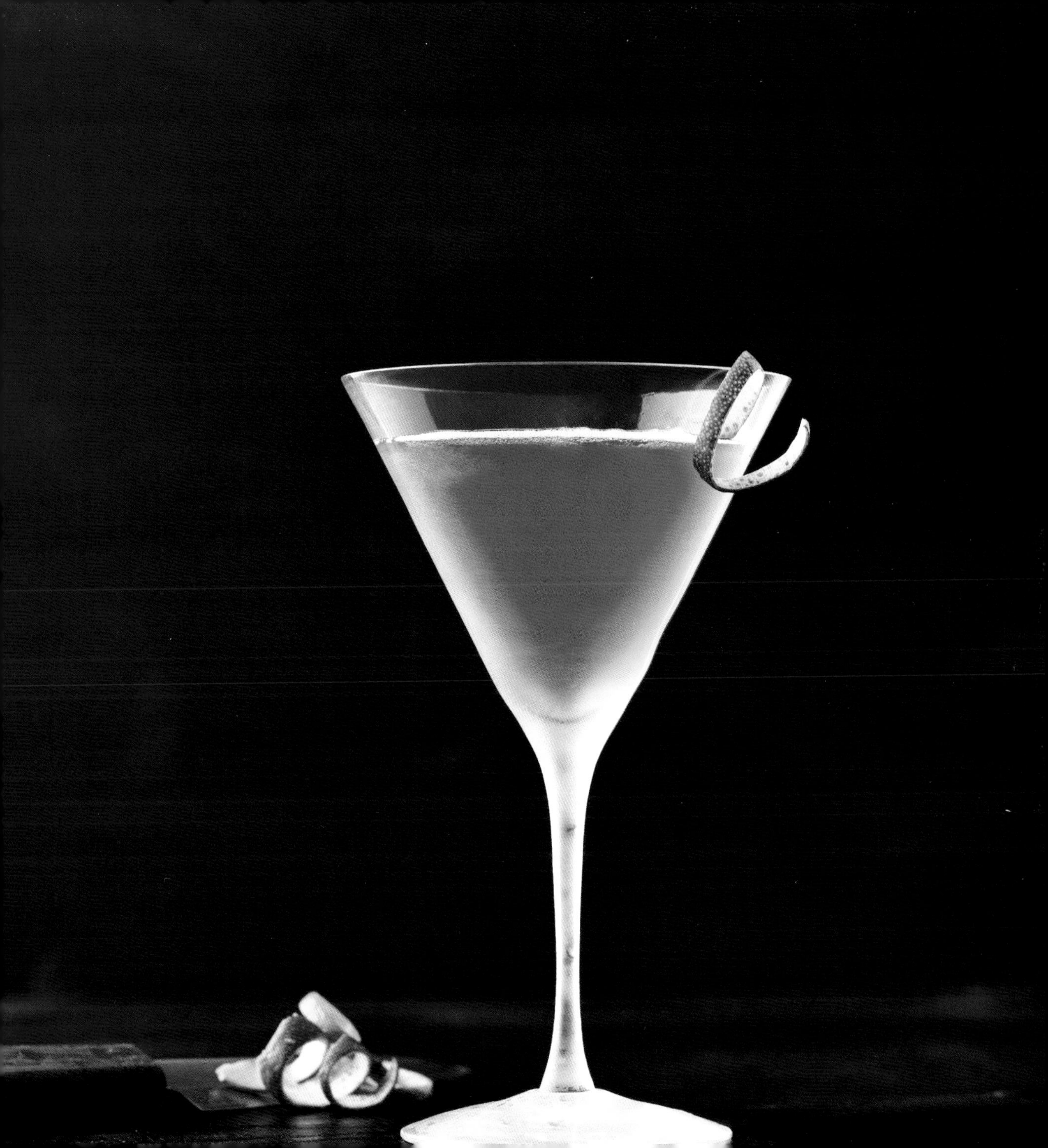

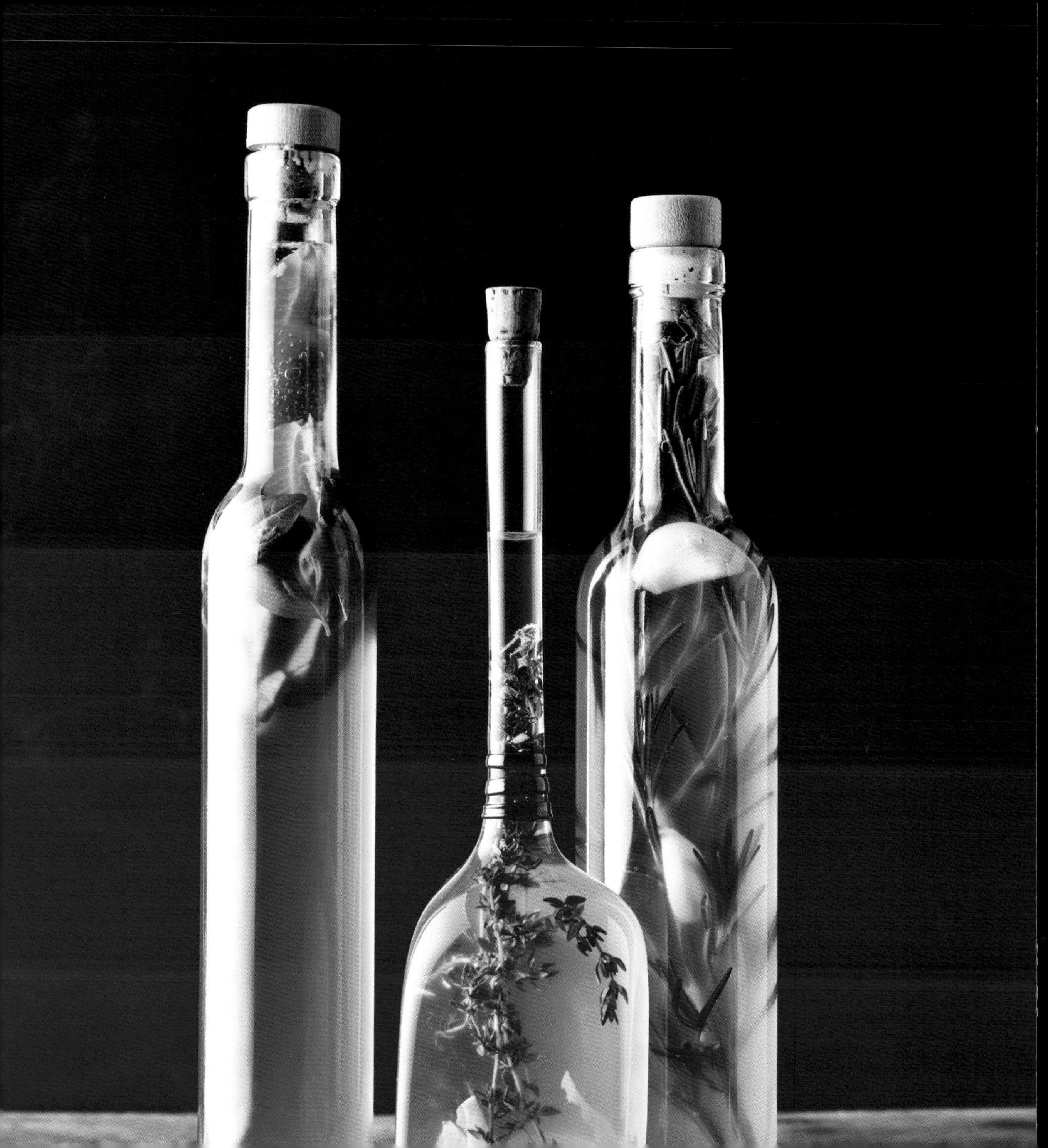

# Kombucha vinegar

Kombucha vinegar is so easy to make! By leaving the kombucha to ferment longer from 4 to 10 weeks, the acidity will increase as the bacteria and yeast continue to eat the sugar and other nutrients. The older the kombucha, the more tart it is. When the kombucha is really sour, it has turned into vinegar. It is slightly milder in taste as the acidity level is 2 percent rather than the 4 to 7 percent in regular vinegar.

## BASIC VINEGAR RECIPE

(For 3–4 liters)

6¼–8½ pints natural kombucha, matured for at least 4 weeks
2 teaspoons raw sugar per 1-pint bottle (2 cups)

**Instructions:** Divide the kombucha into clean 1-pint bottles with tight-fitting lids. Add 2 teaspoons sugar per bottle every second week for 6 weeks (that is, three times). Store at room temperature. After 6 weeks, the vinegar is ready. Flavor with fresh herbs of your choice. The vinegar will last up to 6 months in the fridge.

## FLAVOR SUGGESTIONS

Tip 1:
Strawberry
Fresh basil

Tip 2:
Thinly sliced lemon peel (preferably in spirals)
Fresh thyme

Tip 3:
Garlic cloves (whole)
Fresh rosemary (the whole sprig)

## PASTEURIZING KOMBUCHA VINEGAR

Kombucha vinegar has a long shelf life thanks to its low pH level, but as it continues to ferment and mature over time, the vinegar can develop a less-than-savory taste. Pasteurizing will stop the fermentation process by killing yeast and bacteria. Even if the bacteria are sacrificed, other nutrients like organic acids are retained and the taste is not affected. Pasteurized kombucha vinegar also has less acidity and is healthier than normal, distilled vinegar.

**Instructions:** Heat up kombucha vinegar in a saucepan to 145°F and keep at this temperature for 30 minutes. Take the saucepan off the heat and add a lid. Leave it for 12 to 24 hours. Pour into bottles and add your flavor of choice.

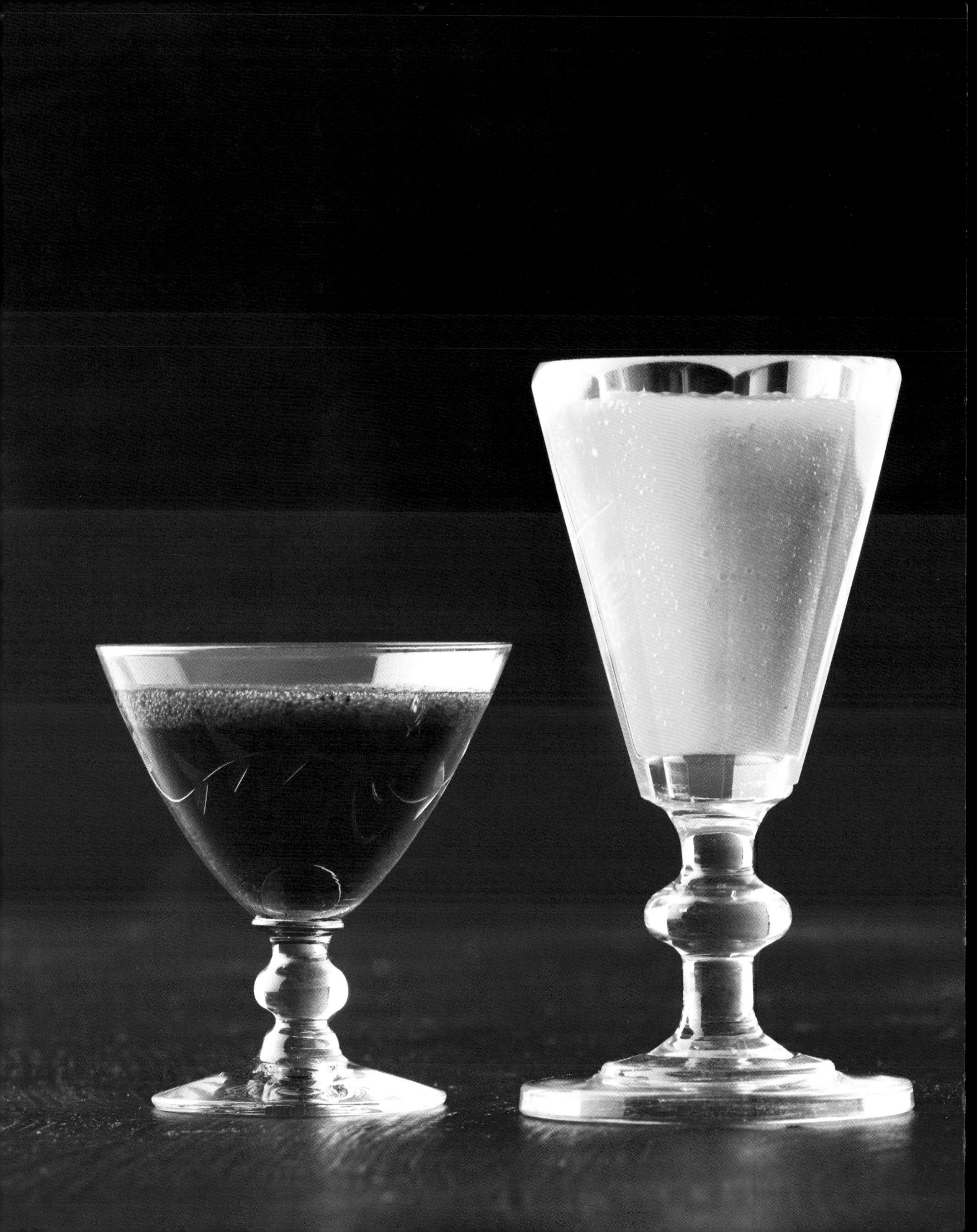

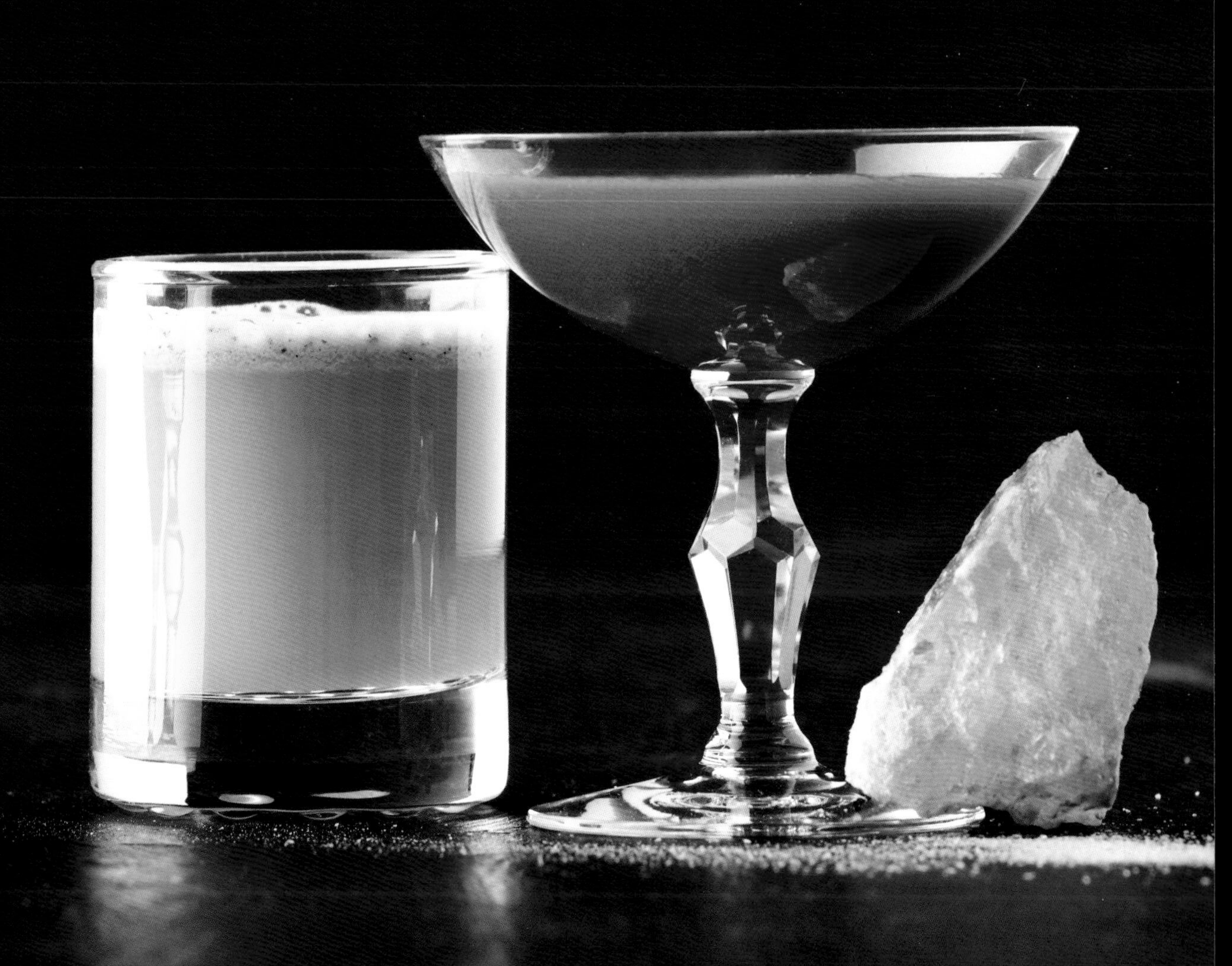

# Around the world in four shots

In tribute to my four favorite places in the world, I have made four kombucha shots, filled to the brim with nutrients that are good for both your gut flora and brain. You're welcome.

## NORDIC LIGHT

2 shots

Blueberries, a superfood from deep in northern Sweden's forests, are packed with nutrients. If you raise your glass to the sun and focus on the dark-blue drink of the heavens, you might even be lucky enough to catch a glimpse of the northern lights.

- 2/5 cup blueberries (frozen are fine)
- 1/2 pear, cut in coarse chunks
- 4/5 cup kombucha
- Pinch of ground cardamom

**Instructions:** Mix the blueberries, pear, kombucha, and cardamom in a blender. Pour into shot glasses and drink.

## BOMBAY SHOT

2 shots

Who hasn't heard of turmeric's anti-inflammatory properties? Truth be told, I'm not totally sold on the flavor of turmeric, but when combined with some mango, magic is created. In one shot, you will be transported to the home of turmeric and mango—India.

- 1 tablespoon turmeric powder
- 2/5 cup mango pieces (frozen are fine)
- 4/5 cup kombucha
- 1/2 lemon
- Black pepper

**Instructions:** Mix the turmeric, mango, and kombucha in a blender. Add the squeezed lemon and a few cracks of pepper. Pour into shot glasses and drink immediately.

## BIG APPLE

2 shots

This gorgeous green shot reminds me of apple martini, which I drank a lot of when I lived in New York. If you want a bit more sweetness, add some drops of honey. If not, I think it tastes great the way it is—and it is also very healthy!

1 large green apple, cut in pieces
¾ inches fresh ginger
Bunch of mint leaves
⅖ cup kombucha
Juice from ½ lime
Pinch of vanilla powder

**Instructions:** Press the apple pieces, ginger, and mint leaves into a juice machine. Add kombucha, lime juice, and vanilla powder. Pour into shot glasses (or why not martini glasses?) and enjoy!

## S(E)OUL SAVIOR

2 shots

This pink shot reminds me of Seoul, where freshly pressed pomegranate juice is extremely popular. Pomegranate is also filled with phenols and antioxidants that, among other things, protect your brain cells. Add a pinch of pink salt from the Himalayas, and your soul will be saved!

1 pomegranate
¼ cup kombucha
Pinch of pink Himalayan salt

**Instructions:** Divide the pomegranate and remove the seeds with a spoon. Press the pomegranate seeds through a juice machine. Add kombucha and Himalayan salt. Pour, close your eyes, and drink.

# EPILOGUE

## *The health revolution begins with you*

With the accelerated epidemic of chronic first-world diseases and mental health disorders, it is clear that something has gone very wrong in our greed for material things and artificial intelligence that keeps us up in the clouds. The new discovery of the bacterial intelligence in our gut gives us hope, because who would have thought that we have our very own pharmaceutical factory deep inside us with trillions of mini-doctors playing a critical role in our brain and mental health? Did you know that the global revenue for antidepressants is projected to reach seventeen billion dollars in 2020? Early research shows that fiber and lactic acid bacteria can have similar effects compared to expensive medicines—without the harmful side effects! This probably won't make pharmaceutical companies happy, but it's great news for the rest. We can protect and strengthen the crown jewel inside our cranium with the help of food, all on our own. Obviously, it also goes without saying that psychological and neurological diseases are extremely complex, where several factors and treatments have to work together, and if you have a diagnosis, you shouldn't stop your medication or other treatments. Instead, view psychobiotic food as a supplement and a preventative health investment. The fact that stress, anxiety, depression, Alzheimer's, Parkinson's, autism, and maybe even ADHD seem to have an important link to bacteria is a revolutionary notion. I hope this drastically reduces the stigma around mental health. Speaking of stress, I'm calmed by the fact that our bacterial superintelligence was discovered in 2008. And yet, despite how rapidly other developments around us have evolved, we still appear to know very little about the biological world closest to us: our own body.

While writing this book, a question kept being asked of me: how is it that you, an IT entrepreneur with a PhD in complex health care systems, are writing a book on gut bacteria and the brain? Well, it's like this: as far back as I can remember, I have been fascinated by all kinds of complex systems. Anything from the cosmos, society, the body, the brain, quantum physics, and our consciousness. Curiosity has led me to different parts of the world via the IT field, research field, and public health; and my ten years inside the walls of health care have had a deep effect on me—sadly, it left painful scars. What worries me is that our health care today is not designed to treat the tsunami of chronic first-world illnesses and mental health problems that are now overwhelming us; rather, it is currently designed to be reactive, specializing at mending and repairing the body when it has already broken. Deeply frustrated over how health care works (or doesn't work), I chose to leave that world for a period of reflection in the Himalayas. However much of a cliché it sounds, I finally had an epiphany: I would use my research skills to translate and promote important groundbreaking knowledge that will help my fellow humans to look after their brains and prevent psychiatric illnesses. Why? So that we can prevent as many people as possible from entering a health-care system that is primarily reactive. This is why you hold this book.

I know—changing learned behavior, trying out a new way of eating, and adopting a totally new lifestyle are some of the hardest things we can do. The first step toward change is to be fully conscious, and in this case about how gut bacteria can strengthen your brain. That is why I want to say a huge congratulations to you for getting through this entire book and the more than four hundred research articles that it is based on. You have taken the first step into the microbiotic health revolution, which is radically changing our views on health and disease. Above all else, you now know how you can, with help of food, protect and strengthen your brain. It is a smart health investment that I hope you and your trillions of bacterial friends will find huge satisfaction in.



"Life is a luminous pause between two mysteries that are yet one."
—*Carl Jung*

# Glossary

**Adrenaline:** A neurotransmitter that's released into the body during stress and puts the body in a state of readiness.

**Autonomous nervous system:** The part of the nervous system that looks after autonomic processes such as breathing, blood circulation, and metabolism.

**Bacteria:** Unicellular organisms that can be found everywhere on earth, even on and in our bodies.

**Butyric acid:** A healthy short-chain fatty acid that can produce different types of healthy bacteria. It has anti-inflammatory properties and can pass through the gut barrier and blood-brain barrier to reach the brain, where it can have several positive effects.

**Cytokines:** A substance that regulates our immune system. There are both inflammatory and anti-inflammatory versions.

**Dopamine:** A neurotransmitter that is released in our brain when we experience something rewarding—also called the brain's *reward drug*. It also controls our voluntary and fine motor movements.

**Enteric nervous system:** The "second brain" consists of the nerve cells in the gut that are reminiscent of our "first brain." It regulates the gut's rhythmic movements, can trigger reflexes, and communicates regularly with the brain in our head.

**Fecal microbiota transplantation (FMT)** *or* **Fecal transplant:** The transplantation of stools from one person to another. It can help restore an unbalanced gut flora and is an effective way to treat many illnesses, such as *C. diff* infections.

**Fermentation:** A chemical process where lactic acid bacteria breaks down carbohydrates and produces lactic acid.

**GABA (gamma-Aminobutyric acid):** A neurotransmitter that calms activity in the brain; a deficiency of GABA is linked to problems like depression and anxiety.

**Gut-brain axis:** The dialogue between the gut and the brain. The state of the gut has an effect on the brain, which can lead to reduced mental health, and in turn the state of mental health has an effect on the gut. Gut bacteria plays a central role in this dialogue as they often pass messages between the gut and brain.

**Gut flora:** The complex ecosystem of microorganisms that live in our gut. As 99 percent of microbiota is in the gut, *gut flora* is often used synonymously with *microbiota*.

**Hippocampus:** An area of the brain that is, among other things, important for memory and mental well-being. In the past it was believed that the brain could not create new nerve cells in adulthood, but now we know that this can occur, but only in the hippocampus. Long-term stress and/or depression can lead to the hippocampus shrinking.

**HPA axis:** Also known as the *stress axis*, this is a system of brain structures and glands that are activated by stress. During stress, signals are sent from the brain to the adrenal glands that it turn release the stress hormones cortisol and adrenaline into the blood. These hormones contribute to the body's fight-or-flight response and equip us to take on stressful situations. However, long term-stress can have negative consequences for the body and brain.

**Human genome:** All genes (around twenty thousand) in the human DNA.

**Immune system:** The body's defense system against intruding viruses, harmful bacteria, harmful parasites, and so on. The immune system consists of, among other things, white blood cells that eat intruders and defense mechanisms like inflammation and fever, which try to burn them away. When the immune system is activated in an improper way, it can cause allergies, chronic inflammation, and autoimmune illnesses. The presence of bacteria in and on our bodies are important for the immune system to develop normally.

**Inulin:** A prebiotic fiber that can be found in onion, roots, green leaves, and others.

**Kimchi:** A tasty, fermented vegetable dish from Korea that is rich in healthy lactic acid bacteria and fiber.

**Kombucha:** A Korean fermented drink that is lightly carbonated and brewed from tea and bacterial culture.

**Lactic acid bacteria:** A group of bacteria that are noted for their ability to convert sugars to lactic acid, which increase the use-by date of fermented food. This group of bacteria can be found in kimchi and kombucha, among others, and many species have been found to have health-promoting effects.

**LPS (lipopolysaccharides):** A mix of fat (lipids) and sugar (saccharides) that give the cell walls of harmful bacteria structure and stability. This substance is toxic for humans and causes strong inflammation when released from inside the bacteria.

**Metabolites:** When an organism breaks down or modifies a molecule, the product is called a metabolite. Depending on what bacteria we have in our gut, different metabolites are produced by the food we eat.

**Microbes or microorganisms:** Describes all unicellular organisms, including bacteria, archaea (bacteria's cousins), protozoa (unicellular "animals"), and yeast (unicellular fungi). Humans have around thirty trillion microbes in and on the body, which can be compared to the roughly thirty trillion human cells in humans.

**Microbiome:** The collected genes found in microorganisms in and on the body. They consist of a hundred times more genes than their own DNA. Sometimes used interchangeably with *microbiota*.

**Microbiota:** Microbiota consists of all microbes that live on your body (e.g., the skin) and in your gut. Sometimes used interchangeably with *microbiome* (see *gut flora*).

**Neuroinflammation:** Inflammation of the brain that doesn't go away but continues over a long period of time. Neuroinflammation appears to be involved in illnesses like depression and Alzheimer's. Inflammatory substances can leak from the gut into the blood and travel all the way to the brain.

**Neurotransmitters:** The substance that nerve cells use to communicate with each other, e.g., glutamate, serotonin, dopamine, noradrenaline, and GABA. Different neurotransmitters have different effects on the brain and can affect mood, wakefulness, concentration, motivation, memory, and movement.

**Noradrenaline:** A substance that activates the body's fight-or-flight response, among other things. It is also important for alertness.

**Oligosaccharides:** Medium-long carbohydrates (saccharides) consisting of three to ten different sugar types that the human gut can't break down. They are consumed by bacteria that in turn produce short-chain fatty acids (such as butyric acid). FOS (fructooligosaccharides), GOS (galactooligosaccharides), and inulin are common types of oligosaccharides.

**Pathogen:** Bacteria, viruses, yeast, etc., that can cause disease are known as *pathogens*. Pathogens are the opposite of probiotics.

**Polyphenol:** A strong antioxidant that gives fruit and vegetables their color, odor. and flavor.

**Prebiotics:** Nutrients that sustain health-promoting bacteria. Fiber is a substance that humans can't break down but that is eaten up by the bacteria in our gut. By eating more of the fiber that provides nutrients for bacteria, you can increase the amount of health-promoting bacteria in your gut.

**Probiotics:** Bacteria that in large enough amounts have health-promoting effects. Lactic acid bacteria is a main player here, but certain types of yeast are also promising candidates.

**Psychobiotics:** Bacteria that have beneficial effects on mental health and the brain, as well as the fiber that feeds these bacteria. Psychobiotics have an effect on the brain that can potentially ease or prevent psychiatric illnesses like depression and anxiety.

**SCOBY:** This stands for *symbiotic culture of bacteria and yeast*—the actual kombucha culture. Also known as *kombucha fungi*, it is actually a thick carpet of biofilm, mainly consisting of the cellulose fiber that stimulates and feeds millions of bacteria in kombucha.

**Serotonin:** A neurotransmitter that regulates worry, anxiety, sleep, pain, and even feelings of being full or hungry. It is also known as the happy hormone. Antidepressants increase the amount of serotonin in your body. It is produced in large amounts in the gut, where it regulates rhythmic movement.

**Short-chain fatty acids:** This is one of the most important metabolites that can affect nerve cells and the hormone system.

**Vagus nerve:** An important nerve that connects the brain with the body's organs. The vagus nerve is a central part of the gut-brain axis as it links the gut with the brain.

# References

## CHAPTER 1

Allen, A. P., Hutch, W., Borre, Y. E., Kennedy, P. J., Temko, A., Boylan, G., ... Clarke, G. (2016). Bifidobacterium longum 1714 as a translational psychobiotic: modulation of stress, electrophysiology and neurocognition in healthy volunteers. *Translational Psychiatry*, 6(11), e939.

Atarashi, K., Tanoue, T., Shima, T., Imaoka, A., Kuwahara, T., Momose, Y., ... Honda, K. (2011). Induction of Colonic Regulatory T Cells by Indigenous Clostridium Species. *Science*, 331(6015), 337–341.

Baquero, F., & Nombela, C. (2012). The microbiome as a human organ. *Clinical Microbiology and Infection*, 18(SUPPL. 4), 2–4.

Bowden, M. (July 2012). The Measured Man. *The Atlantic*. Accessed from https://www.theatlantic.com/magazine/archive/2012/07/the-measured-man/309018/

Clarke, G., Stilling, R. M., Kennedy, P. J., Stanton, C., Cryan, J. F., & Dinan, T. G. (2014). Minireview: Gut Microbiota: The Neglected Endocrine Organ. *Molecular Endocrinology*, 28(8), 1221–1238.

Eme, L., Spang, A., Lombard, J., Stairs, C. W., & Ettema, T. J. G. (2017). Archaea and the origin of eukaryotes. *Nature Reviews Microbiology*, 15(12), 711–723.

Engelhardt, B., Carare, R. O., Bechmann, I., Flügel, A., Laman, J. D., & Weller, R. O. (2016). Vascular, glial, and lymphatic immune gateways of the central nervous system. *Acta neuropathologica*, 132(3), 317–38.

Evans, J. M., Morris, L. S., & Marchesi, J. R. (2013). The gut microbiome: The role of a virtual organ in the endocrinology of the host. *Journal of Endocrinology*, 218(3).

Fierer, N., Hamady, M., Lauber, C. L., & Knight, R. (2008). The influence of sex, handedness, and washing on the diversity of hand surface bacteria. *Proceedings of the National Academy of Sciences of the United States of America*, 105(46), 17994–9.

Fischer, S. (2012, november). What Lives in Your Belly Button? Study Finds “Rain Forest” of Species. *National Geographic*. Accessed from https://news.nationalgeographic.com/news/2012/11/121114-belly-button-bacteria-science-health-dunn/

Gilbert, J. A., & Neufeld, J. D. (2014). Life in a World without Microbes. *PLoS Biology*, 12(12), e1002020.

Goehler, L. E., Park, S. M., Opitz, N., Lyte, M., & Gaykema, R. P. A. (2008). Campylobacter jejuni infection increases anxiety-like behavior in the holeboard: Possible anatomical substrates for viscerosensory modulation of exploratory behavior. *Brain, Behavior, and Immunity*, 22(3), 354–366.

Goodrich, J. K., Davenport, E. R., Beaumont, M., Jackson, M. A., Knight, R., Ober, C., ... Ley, R. E. (2016). Genetic Determinants of the Gut Microbiome in UK Twins. *Cell Host & Microbe*, 19(5), 731–43.

Goodrich, J. K., Waters, J. L., Poole, A. C., Sutter, J. L., Koren, O., Blekhman, R., ... Ley, R. E. (2014). Human genetics shape the gut microbiome. *Cell*, 159(4), 789–99.

Hulcr, J., Latimer, A. M., Henley, J. B., Rountree, N. R., Fierer, N., Lucky, A., ... Dunn, R. R. (2012). A Jungle in There: Bacteria in Belly Buttons are Highly Diverse, but Predictable. *PLoS ONE*, 7(11), e47712.

Huttenhower, C., Gevers, D., Knight, R., Abubucker, S., Badger, J. H., Chinwalla, A. T., ... White, O. (2012). Structure, function and diversity of the healthy human microbiome. *Nature*, 486(7402), 207–214.

Janssen, A. W. F., & Kersten, S. (2015). The role of the gut microbiota in metabolic health. *FASEB Journal*, 29(8), 3111–3123.

Jumpertz, R., Le, D. S., Turnbaugh, P. J., Trinidad, C., Bogardus, C., Gordon, J. I., & Krakoff, J. (2011). Energy-balance studies reveal associations between gut microbes, caloric load, and nutrient absorption in humans. *American Journal of Clinical Nutrition*, 94(1), 58–65.

Karimi, K., Inman, M. D., Bienenstock, J., & Forsythe, P. (2009). Lactobacillus reuteri-induced regulatory T cells protect against an allergic airway response in mice. *American Journal of Respiratory and Critical Care Medicine*, 179(3), 186–193.

Koliada, A., Syzenko, G., Moseiko, V., Budovska, L., Puchkov, K., Perederiy, V., … Vaiserman, A. (2017). Association between body mass index and Firmicutes/Bacteroidetes ratio in an adult Ukrainian population. *BMC Microbiology*, 17(1), 120.

Luckey, T. D. (1972). Introduction to intestinal microecology. *American Journal of Clinical Nutrition*, 25(12), 1292–1294.

Magnúsdóttir, S., Ravcheev, D., de Crécy-Lagard, V., & Thiele, I. (2015). Systematic genome assessment of B-vitamin biosynthesis suggests co-operation among gut microbes. *Frontiers in Genetics*, 6, 148.

Maier, L., Pruteanu, M., Kuhn, M., Zeller, G., Telzerow, A., Anderson, E. E., Brochado, A. R., Fernandez, K. C., Dose, H., Mori, H., Patil, K. R., Bork, P., Typas, A. (2018). Extensive impact of non-antibiotic drugs on human gut bacteria, *Nature*, 555 (7698), 623–628.

McCourtie, J., & Douglas, L. J. (1984). Relationship between cell surface composition, adherence, and virulence of *Candida albicans. Infection and Immunity*, 45(1), 6–12.

McFall-Ngai, M. (2007). Adaptive immunity: Care for the community. *Nature*, 445(7124), 153–153.

Messaoudi, M., Lalonde, R., Violle, N., Javelot, H., Desor, D., Nejdi, A., … Cazaubiel, J.-M. (2011). Assessment of psychotropic-like properties of a probiotic formulation (Lactobacillus helveticus R0052 and Bifidobacterium longum R0175) in rats and human subjects. *British Journal of Nutrition*, 105(5), 755–764.

Neuman, H., Debelius, J. W., Knight, R., & Koren, O. (2015). Microbial endocrinology: the interplay between the microbiota and the endocrine system. *FEMS Microbiology Reviews*, 39(4), 509–521.

Perez-Muñoz, M. E., Arrieta, M.-C., Ramer-Tait, A. E., & Walter, J. (2017). A critical assessment of the "sterile womb" and "in utero colonization" hypotheses: implications for research on the pioneer infant microbiome. *Microbiome*, 5(1), 48.

Pinto-Sanchez, M. I., Hall, G. B., Ghajar, K., Nardelli, A., Bolino, C., Lau, J. T., … Bercik, P. (2017). Probiotic Bifidobacterium longum NCC3001 Reduces Depression Scores and Alters Brain Activity: A Pilot Study in Patients With Irritable Bowel Syndrome. *Gastroenterology*, 77(0), 1282–1289.

Qin, J., Li, R., Raes, J., Arumugam, M., Burgdorf, K. S., Manichanh, C., … Wang, J. (2010). A human gut microbial gene catalogue established by metagenomic sequencing. *Nature*, 464(7285), 59–65.

Sender, R., Fuchs, S., & Milo, R. (2016). Revised Estimates for the Number of Human and Bacteria Cells in the Body. *PLOS Biology*, 14(8), e1002533.

Wallace, T. D., Bradley, S., Buckley, N. D., & Green-Johnson, J. M. (2003). Interactions of lactic acid bacteria with human intestinal epithelial cells: effects on cytokine production. *Journal of Food Protection*, 66(3), 466–72.

Wang, Z., & Nakayama, T. (2010). Inflammation, a link between obesity and cardiovascular disease. *Mediators of Inflammation*, 2010, 535918.

## CHAPTER 2

Al-Sadi, R., Boivin, M., & Ma, T. (2009). Mechanism of cytokine modulation of epithelial tight junction barrier. *Frontiers in Bioscience* (Landmark edition), 14, 2765–78.

Alcock J., Maley C.C., Actipis C.A. (2014) Is eating behavior manipulated by the gastrointestinal microbiota? Evolutionary pressures and potential mechanisms. *Bioessays*. 2014 Oct;36 (10):940-9.

Almy, T. P., Kern, F., & Tulin, M. (1949). Alterations in Colonic Function in Man Under Stress: II. Experimental Production of Sigmoid Spasm in Healthy Persons. *Gastroenterology*, 12(3), 425–436.

Bailey, M. T., Lubach, G. R., & Coe, C. L. (2004). Prenatal stress alters bacterial colonization of the gut in infant monkeys. *Journal of Pediatric Gastroenterology and Nutrition*, 38(4), 414–421.

Bleich, H. L., Moore, M. J., Roth, J., LeRoith, D., Shiloach, J., Rosenzweig, J. L., ... Havrankova, J. (1982). The Evolutionary Origins of Hormones, Neurotransmitters, and Other Extracellular Chemical Messengers. *New England Journal of Medicine*, 306(9), 523–527.

Bonaz, B., Bazin, T., & Pellissier, S. (2018). The vagus nerve at the interface of the microbiota-gut-brain axis. *Frontiers in Neuroscience*. Frontiers Media SA.

Bravo, J. A., Forsythe, P., Chew, M. V, Escaravage, E., Savignac, H. M., Dinan, T. G., ... Cryan, J. F. (2011). Ingestion of Lactobacillus strain regulates emotional behavior and central GABA receptor expression in a mouse via the vagus nerve. *Proceedings of the National Academy of Sciences of the United States of America*, 108(38), 16050–5.

Canani, R. B., Costanzo, M. Di, Leone, L., Pedata, M., Meli, R., & Calignano, A. (2011). Potential beneficial effects of butyrate in intestinal and extraintestinal diseases. *World Journal of Gastroenterology*, 17(12), 1519–28.

De Filippo, C., Cavalieri, D., Di Paola, M., Ramazzotti, M., Poullet, J. B., Massart, S., ... Lionetti, P. (2010). Impact of diet in shaping gut microbiota revealed by a comparative study in children from Europe and rural Africa. *Proceedings of the National Academy of Sciences of the United States of America*, 107(33), 14691–6.

De Palma, G., Blennerhassett, P., Lu, J., Deng, Y., Park, A. J., Green, W., ... Bercik, P. (2015). Microbiota and host determinants of behavioural phenotype in maternally separated mice. *Nature Communications*, 6(1), 7735.

Desbonnet, L., Garrett, L., Clarke, G., Bienenstock, J., & Dinan, T. G. (2008). The probiotic Bifidobacteria infantis: An assessment of potential antidepressant properties in the rat. *Journal of Psychiatric Research*, 43(2), 164–174.

Dinan, T. G., & Cryan, J. F. (March 1, 2017). The Microbiome-Gut-Brain Axis in Health and Disease. *Gastroenterology Clinics of North America*. Elsevier.

Dinan, T. G., Stilling, R. M., Stanton, C., & Cryan, J. F. (2015). Collective unconscious: How gut microbes shape human behavior. *Journal of Psychiatric Research*, 63, 1–9.

Ekman, P. (1992). An argument for basic emotions. Cognition and Emotion, 6(3–4), 169–200.

Endo, T., Minami, M., Hirafuji, M., Ogawa, T., Akita, K., Nemoto, M., ... Parvez, S. H. (2000). Neurochemistry and neuropharmacology of emesis — the role of serotonin. *Toxicology*, 153(1–3), 189–201.

Engelhardt, B., Carare, R. O., Bechmann, I., Flügel, A., Laman, J. D., & Weller, R. O. (2016). Vascular, glial, and lymphatic immune gateways of the central nervous system. *Acta Neuropathologica*, 132(3), 317–38.

Foley, J. O., & DuBois, F. S. (1937). Quantitative studies of the vagus nerve in the cat. I. The ratio of sensory to motor fibers. *Journal of Comparative Neurology*, 67(1), 49–67.

Fond, G., Loundou, A., Hamdani, N., Boukouaci, W., Dargel, A., Oliveira, J., ... Boyer, L. (2014). Anxiety and depression comorbidities in irritable bowel syndrome (IBS): a systematic review and meta-analysis. *European Archives of Psychiatry and Clinical neuroscience*, 264(8), 651–660.

Forsyth, C. B., Shannon, K. M., Kordower, J. H., Voigt, R. M., Shaikh, M., Jaglin, J. A., ... Keshavarzian, A. (2011). Increased intestinal permeability correlates with sigmoid mucosa alpha-synuclein staining and endotoxin exposure markers in early Parkinson's disease. *PLoS ONE*, 6(12).

Freestone, P. P. E., Sandrini, S. M., Haigh, R. D., & Lyte, M. (2008). Microbial endocrinology: how stress influences susceptibility to infection. *Trends in Microbiology*, 16(2), 55–64.

Furness, J. B., Rivera, L. R., Cho, H.-J., Bravo, D. M., & Callaghan, B. (2013). The gut as a sensory organ. *Nature Reviews Gastroenterology & Hepatology*, 1010(1212), 729–740.

Furness, J. B., & Stebbing, M. J. (2018, February 1). The first brain: Species comparisons and evolutionary implications for the enteric and central nervous systems. *Neurogastroenterology and Motility*. Wiley/ Blackwell (10.1111).

Garvey, M., Noyes, R., & Yates, W. (1990). Frequency of Constipation in Major Depression: Relationship to Other Clinical Variables. *Psychosomatics*, 31(2), 204–206.

Gershon, M. D. (2013). 5-Hydroxytryptamine (serotonin) in the gastrointestinal tract. *Current Opinion in Endocrinology, Diabetes, and Obesity*, 20(1), 14–21.

Govindarajan, N., Agis-Balboa, R. C., Walter, J., Sananbenesi, F., & Fischer, A. (2011). Sodium butyrate improves memory function in an Alzheimer's disease mouse model when administered at an advanced stage of disease progression. *Journal of Alzheimer's Disease*, 26(1), 187–197.

Guan, Z., & Fang, J. (2006). Peripheral immune activation by lipopolysaccharide decreases neurotrophins in the cortex and hippocampus in rats. *Brain, Behavior, and Immunity*, 20(1), 64–71.

Guo, S., Al-Sadi, R., Said, H. M., & Ma, T. Y. (2013). Lipopolysaccharide causes an increase in intestinal tight junction permeability in vitro and in vivo by inducing enterocyte membrane expression and localization of TLR-4 and CD14. *American Journal of Pathology*, 182(2), 375–87.

Hanson, C. S., Outhred, T., Brunoni, A. R., Malhi, G. S., & Kemp, A. H. (2013). The impact of escitalopram on vagally mediated cardiovascular function to stress and the moderating effects of vigorous physical activity: a randomized controlled treatment study in healthy participants. *Frontiers in Physiology*, 4, 259.

Howland, R. H. (2014). Vagus Nerve Stimulation. Current behavioral neuroscience reports, 1(2), 64–73.

Kitamoto, S., Nagao-Kitamoto, H., Kuffa, P., & Kamada, N. (2016). Regulation of virulence: the rise and fall of gastrointestinal pathogens. *Journal of Gastroenterology*, 51(3), 195–205.



Lam, D. D., Garfield, A. S., Marston, O. J., Shaw, J., & Heisler, L. K. (2010). Brain serotonin system in the coordination of food intake and body weight. *Pharmacology Biochemistry and Behavior*, 97(1), 84–91.

Larson, E. T., & Summers, C. H. (2001). Serotonin reverses dominant social status. *Behavioural Brain Research*, 121(1–2), 95–102.

Lee, J., Lee, Y., Yuk, D., Choi, D., Ban, S., Oh, K., & Hong, J. (2008). Neuro-inflammation induced by lipopolysaccharide causes cognitive impairment through enhancement of beta-amyloid generation. *Journal of Neuroinflammation*, 5(1), 37.

Ley, R. E., Lozupone, C. A., Hamady, M., Knight, R., & Gordon, J. I. (2008). Worlds within worlds: evolution of the vertebrate gut microbiota. *Nature Reviews Microbiology*, 6(10), 776–788.

Ley, R. E., Turnbaugh, P. J., Klein, S., & Gordon, J. I. (2006). Microbial ecology: Human gut microbes associated with obesity. *Nature*, 444(7122), 1022–1023.

Maier, L., Pruteanu, M., Kuhn, M., Zeller, G., Telzerow, A., Anderson, E. E., Brochado, A. R., Fernandez, K. C., Dose, H., Mori, H., Patil, K. R., Bork, P., Typas, A. (2018). Extensive impact of non-antibiotic drugs on human gut bacteria, *Nature*, 555 (7698), 623–628.

Maloof, A. C., Porter, S. M., Moore, J. L., Dudás, F. Ö., Bowring, S. A., Higgins, J. A., ... Eddy, M. P. (2010). The earliest Cambrian record of animals and ocean geochemical change. *Bulletin of the Geological Society of America*, 122(11–12), 1731–1774.

Mayer, E. (2016). *The Mind-Gut Connection: How the Hidden Conversation within Our Bodies Impacts Our Mood, Our Choices, and Our Overall Health.* New York: HarperCollins.

Mayer, E. A. (2011). Gut feelings: the emerging biology of gut–brain communication. *Nature Reviews Neuroscience*, 12(8), 453–466.

Miller, A. H., Haroon, E., Raison, C. L., & Felger, J. C. (2013). Cytokine targets in the brain: impact on neurotransmitters and neurocircuits. *Depression and Anxiety*, 30(4), 297–306.

Miller, M. B., & Bassler, B. L. (2001). Quorum Sensing in Bacteria. *Annual Review of Microbiology*, 55(1), 165–199.

Miyauchi, E., Morita, H., & Tanabe, S. (2009). Lactobacillus rhamnosus alleviates intestinal barrier dysfunction in part by increasing expression of zonula occludens-1 and myosin light-chain kinase in vivo. *Journal of Dairy Science*, 92(6), 2400–8.

Morrison, D. J., & Preston, T. (2016). Formation of short chain fatty acids by the gut microbiota and their impact on human metabolism. *Gut Microbes*, 7(3), 189–200.

Murry, A. C., Hinton, A., & Morrison, H. (2004). Inhibition of growth of Escherichia coli, Salmonella typhimurium, and Clostridia perfringens on chicken feed media by Lactobacillus salivarius and Lactobacillus plantarum. *International Journal of Poultry Science*, 3(9), 603–607.

Nagpal, R., Kumar, A., Kumar, M., Behare, P. V., Jain, S., & Yadav, H. (2012). Probiotics, their health benefits and applications for developing healthier foods: a review. *FEMS Microbiology Letters*, 334(1), 1–15.

Perry, R. J., Peng, L., Barry, N. A., Cline, G. W., Zhang, D., Cardone, R. L., ... Shulman, G. I. (2016). Acetate mediates a microbiome–brain–β-cell axis to promote metabolic syndrome. *Nature*, 534(7606), 213–217.

Psichas, A., Reimann, F., & Gribble, F. M. (March 2, 2015). Gut chemosensing mechanisms. *Journal of Clinical Investigation*. American Society for Clinical Investigation.

Réus, G. Z., Fries, G. R., Stertz, L., Badawy, M., Passos, I. C., Barichello, T., ... Quevedo, J. (2015). The role of inflammation and microglial activation in the pathophysiology of psychiatric disorders. *Neuroscience*, 300, 141–154.

Rios, A. C., Maurya, P. K., Pedrini, M., Zeni-Graiff, M., Asevedo, E., Mansur, R. B., ... Brietzke, E. (2017). Microbiota abnormalities and the therapeutic potential of probiotics in the treatment of mood disorders. *Reviews in the Neurosciences*, 28(7), 739–749.

Rozengurt, E., & Sternini, C. (2007). Taste receptor signaling in the mammalian gut. *Current Opinion in Pharmacology*, 7(6), 557–562.

Ruffoli, R., Giorgi, F. S., Pizzanelli, C., Murri, L., Paparelli, A., & Fornai, F. (2011). The chemical neuroanatomy of vagus nerve stimulation. *Journal of Chemical Neuroanatomy*, 42(4), 288–296.

Schmidt, K., Cowen, P. J., Harmer, C. J., Tzortzis, G., Errington, S., & Burnet, P. W. J. (2015). Prebiotic intake reduces the waking cortisol response and alters emotional bias in healthy volunteers. *Psychopharmacology*, 232(10), 1793–1801.

Sikander, A., Rana, S. V., & Prasad, K. K. (2009). Role of serotonin in gastrointestinal motility and irritable bowel syndrome. *Clinica Chimica Acta*, 403(1–2), 47–55.

Stevens, B. R., Goel, R., Seungbum, K., Richards, E. M., Holbert, R. C., Pepine, C. J., & Raizada, M. K. (2017). Increased human intestinal barrier permeability plasma biomarkers zonulin and FABP2 correlated with plasma LPS and altered gut microbiome in anxiety or depression. *Gut*.

Stilling, R. M., Bordenstein, S. R., Dinan, T. G., & Cryan, J. F. (2014). Friends with social benefits: host-microbe interactions as a driver of brain evolution and development? *Frontiers in Cellular and Infection Microbiology*, 4, 147.

Symonds, E. L., O'Mahony, C., Lapthorne, S., O'Mahony, D., Sharry, J. Mac, O'Mahony, L., & Shanahan, F. (2012). Bifidobacterium infantis 35624 protects against Salmonella-induced reductions in digestive enzyme activity in mice by attenuation of the host inflammatory response. *Clinical and Translational Gastroenterology*, 3(5), e15–e15.

Turnbaugh, P. J., Hamady, M., Yatsunenko, T., Cantarel, B. L., Duncan, A., Ley, R. E., ... Gordon, J. I. (2009). A core gut microbiome in obese and lean twins. *Nature*, 457(7228), 480–484.

Turnbaugh, P. J., Ridaura, V. K., Faith, J. J., Rey, F. E., Knight, R., & Gordon, J. I. (2009). The effect of diet on the human gut microbiome: a metagenomic analysis in humanized gnotobiotic mice. *Science Translational Medicine*, 1(6), 6ra14.

Vanuytsel, T., van Wanrooy, S., Vanheel, H., Vanormelingen, C., Verschueren, S., Houben, E., ... Tack, J. (2014). Psychological stress and corticotropin-releasing hormone increase intestinal permeability in humans by a mast cell-dependent mechanism. *Gut*, 63(8), 1293–9.

Vlisidou, I., Lyte, M., van Diemen, P. M., Hawes, P., Monaghan, P., Wallis, T. S., & Stevens, M. P. (2004). The neuroendocrine stress hormone norepinephrine augments Escherichia coli O157:H7-induced enteritis and adherence in a bovine ligated ileal loop model of infection. *Infection and immunity*, 72(9), 5446–51.

Walker, E. A., Katon, W. J., Jemelka, R. P., & Roy-Byrne, P. P. (1992). Comorbidity of gastrointestinal complaints, depression, and anxiety in the epidemiologic catchment area (ECA) study. *American Journal of Medicine*, 92(1), S26–S30.

Welgan, P., Meshkinpour, H., & Beeler, M. (1988). Effect of anger on colon motor and myoelectric activity in irritable bowel syndrome. *Gastroenterology*, 94(5), 1150–1156.

Yano, J. M., Yu, K., Donaldson, G. P., Shastri, G. G., Ann, P., Ma, L., ... Hsiao, E. Y. (2015). Indigenous Bacteria from the Gut Microbiota Regulate Host Serotonin Biosynthesis. *Cell*, 161(2), 264–276.

Zhang, R., Miller, R. G., Gascon, R., Champion, S., Katz, J., Lancero, M., . . . McGrath, M. S. (2009). Circulating endotoxin and systemic immune activation in sporadic amyotrophic lateral sclerosis (sALS). *Journal of Neuroimmunology*, 206(1–2), 121–4.

Zhu, B., Wang, Z. G., Ding, J., Liu, N., Wang, D. M., Ding, L. C., & Yang, C. (2014). Chronic lipopolysaccharide exposure induces cognitive dysfunction without affecting BDNF expression in the rat hippocampus. *Experimental and Therapeutic Medicine*, 7(3), 750–754.

## CHAPTER 3



Aarsland, D., Påhlhagen, S., Ballard, C. G., Ehrt, U., & Svenningsson, P. (2012). Depression in Parkinson disease—epidemiology, mechanisms and management. *Nature Reviews Neurology*, 8(1), 35–47.

Aarts, E., Ederveen, T. H. A., Naaijen, J., Zwiers, M. P., Boekhorst, J., Timmerman, H. M., ... Arias Vasquez, A. (2017). Gut microbiome in ADHD and its relation to neural reward anticipation. *PLOS ONE*, 12(9), e0183509.

Adams, J. B., Johansen, L. J., Powell, L. D., Quig, D., & Rubin, R. A. (2011). Gastrointestinal flora and gastrointestinal status in children with autism – comparisons to typical children and correlation with autism severity. *BMC Gastroenterology*, 11(1), 22.

Akbari, E., Asemi, Z., Kakhaki, R. D., Bahmani, F., Kouchaki, E., Tamtaji, O. R., ... Salami, M. (2016). Effect of probiotic supplementation on cognitive function and metabolic status in Alzheimer's disease: A randomized, double-blind and controlled trial. *Frontiers in Aging Neuroscience*, 8(NOV).

Allen, A. P., Hutch, W., Borre, Y. E., Kennedy, P. J., Temko, A., Boylan, G., ... Clarke, G. (2016). Bifidobacterium longum 1714 as a translational psychobiotic: modulation of stress, electrophysiology and neurocognition in healthy volunteers. *Translational Psychiatry*, 6(11), e939.

American Academy of Pediatrics. (2012). Breastfeeding and the Use of Human Milk. Pediatrics (Vol. 19).

American Foundation for Suicide Prevention. (2017). Suicide Statistics. https://afsp.org/about-suicide/suicide-statistics/.

American Psychiatric Association. (2017). What is Depression? https://www.psychiatry.org/patients-families/depression/what-is-depression.

Angelis, M. De, Piccolo, M., Vannini, L., Siragusa, S., Giacomo, A. De, Serrazzanetti, D. I., ... Francavilla, R. (2013). Fecal Microbiota and Metabolome of Children with Autism and Pervasive Developmental Disorder Not Otherwise Specified. *PLOS ONE*, 8(10), e76993.

Arentsen, T., Qian, Y., Gkotzis, S., Femenia, T., Wang, T., Udekwu, K., ... Diaz Heijtz, R. (2016). The bacterial peptidoglycan-sensing molecule Pglyrp2 modulates brain development and behavior. *Molecular Psychiatry*, 22(August), 1–10.

Ascherio, A., Zhang, S. M., Hernán, M. A., Kawachi, I., Colditz, G. A., Speizer, F. E., & Willett, W. C. (2001). Prospective study of caffeine consumption and risk of Parkinson's disease in men and women. *Annals of Neurology*, 50(1), 56–63.

Atladóttir, H. Ó., Henriksen, T. B., Schendel, D. E., & Parner, E. T. (2012). Autism after infection, febrile episodes, and antibiotic use during pregnancy: an exploratory study. *Pediatrics*, 130(6), e1447-54.

Azad, M. B., Konya, T., Maughan, H., Guttman, D. S., Field, C. J., Chari, R. S., ... CHILD Study Investigators. (2013). Gut microbiota of healthy Canadian infants: profiles by mode of delivery and infant diet at 4 months. *CMAJ : Canadian Medical Association journal = journal de l'Association medicale canadienne*, 185(5), 385–94.

Bailey, M. T., & Coe, C. L. (1999). Maternal separation disrupts the integrity of the intestinal microflora in infant rhesus monkeys. *Developmental Psychobiology*, 35(2), 146–155.

Bailey, M. T., Lubach, G. R., & Coe, C. L. (2004). Prenatal stress alters bacterial colonization of the gut in infant monkeys. *Journal of Pediatric Gastroenterology and Nutrition*, 38(4), 414–421.

Bambling, M. et al. (2017) A combination of probiotics and magnesium orotate attenuate depression in a small SSRI resistant cohort: an intestinal anti-inflammatory response is suggested. Springer International Publishing, 2017

Barichella, M., Pacchetti, C., Bolliri, C., Cassani, E., Iorio, L., Pusani, C., ... Cereda, E. (2016). Probiotics and prebiotic fiber for constipation associated with Parkinson disease. *Neurology*, 87(12), 1274–1280.

Bell, J. A., Kivimäki, M., Bullmore, E. T., Steptoe, A., Bullmore, E., Vértes, P. E., ... Carvalho, L. A. (2017). Repeated exposure to systemic inflammation and risk of new depressive symptoms among older adults. *Translational Psychiatry*, 7(8), e1208.

Bercik, P., Denou, E., Collins, J., Jackson, W., Lu, J., Jury, J., ... Collins, S. M. (2011). The Intestinal Microbiota Affect Central Levels of Brain-Derived Neurotropic Factor and Behavior in Mice. *Gastroenterology*, 141(2), 599–609.e3.

Bonfili, L., Cecarini, V., Berardi, S., Scarpona, S., Suchodolski, J. S., Nasuti, C., ... Eleuteri, A. M. (2017). Microbiota modulation counteracts Alzheimer's disease progression influencing neuronal proteolysis and gut hormones plasma levels. *Scientific Reports*, 7(1), 2426.

Bravo, J. A., Forsythe, P., Chew, M. V, Escaravage, E., Savignac, H. M., Dinan, T. G., ... Cryan, J. F. (2011). Ingestion of Lactobacillus strain regulates emotional behavior and central GABA receptor expression in a mouse via the vagus nerve. *Proceedings of the National Academy of Sciences of the United States of America*, 108(38), 16050–5.

Buescher, A. V. S., Cidav, Z., Knapp, M., & Mandell, D. S. (2014). Costs of Autism Spectrum Disorders in the United Kingdom and the United States. *JAMA Pediatrics*, 168(8), 721.

BrainTest. Dementia Statistics – U.S. & Worldwide Stats. https://braintest.com/dementia-stats-u-s-worldwide/.

Buffington, S. A., Di Prisco, G. V., Auchtung, T. A., Ajami, N. J., Petrosino, J. F., & Costa-Mattioli, M. (2016). Microbial Reconstitution Reverses Maternal Diet-Induced Social and Synaptic Deficits in Offspring. *Cell*, 165(7), 1762–1775.

Burrus, C. J. (2012). A biochemical rationale for the interaction between gastrointestinal yeast and autism. *Medical Hypotheses*, 79(6), 784–5.

Byers, A. L., & Yaffe, K. (2011). Depression and risk of developing dementia. *Nature Reviews Neurology*, 7(6), 323–331.

Cattaneo, A., Cattane, N., Galluzzi, S., Provasi, S., Lopizzo, N., Festari, C., ... Frisoni, G. B. (2017). Association of brain amyloidosis with pro-inflammatory gut bacterial taxa and peripheral inflammation markers in cognitively impaired elderly. *Neurobiology of Aging*, 49, 60–68.

Centers for Disease Control and Prevention. (2018). Data and Statistics about ADHD. https://www.cdc.gov/ncbddd/adhd/data.html.

Cermak, S. A., Curtin, C., & Bandini, L. G. (2010). Food selectivity and sensory sensitivity in children with autism spectrum disorders. *Journal of the American Dietetic Association*, 110(2), 238.

Chen, J. jun, Zhou, C. juan, Zheng, P., Cheng, K., Wang, H. yang, Li, J., ... Xie, P. (2017). Differential urinary metabolites related with the severity of major depressive disorder. *Behavioural Brain Research*, 332(April), 280–287.

Cong, X., Henderson, W. A., Graf, J., & McGrath, J. M. (2015). Early Life Experience and Gut Microbiome: The Brain-Gut-Microbiota Signaling System. *Advances in Neonatal Care: Official Journal of the National Association of Neonatal Nurses*, 15(5), 314-23–2.

Connolly, N., Anixt, J., Manning, P., Ping-I Lin, D., Marsolo, K. A., & Bowers, K. (2016). Maternal metabolic risk factors for autism spectrum disorder—An analysis of electronic medical records and linked birth data. *Autism Research*, 9(8), 829–837.

Costantini, L., Molinari, R., Farinon, B., & Merendino, N. (2017). Impact of Omega-3 Fatty Acids on the Gut Microbiota. *International Journal of Molecular Sciences*, 18(12).

Cowan, T. E., Palmnäs, M. S. A., Yang, J., Bomhof, M. R., Ardell, K. L., Reimer, R. A., ... Shearer, J. (2014). Chronic coffee consumption in the diet-induced obese rat: impact on gut microbiota and serum metabolomics. *Journal of Nutritional Biochemistry,* 25(4), 489–495.

Curran, E. A., Dalman, C., Kearney, P. M., Kenny, L. C., Cryan, J. F., Dinan, T. G., & Khashan, A. S. (2015). Association Between Obstetric Mode of Delivery and Autism Spectrum Disorder. *JAMA Psychiatry*, 72(9), 935.



De la Fuente, M., Franchi, L., Araya, D., Díaz-Jiménez, D., Olivares, M., Álvarez-Lobos, M., ... Hermoso, M. A. (2014). Escherichia coli isolates from inflammatory bowel diseases patients survive in macrophages and activate NLRP3 inflammasome. *International Journal of Medical Microbiology*, 304(3–4), 384–392.

De Palma, G., Blennerhassett, P., Lu, J., Deng, Y., Park, A. J., Green, W., ... Bercik, P. (2015). Microbiota and host determinants of behavioural phenotype in maternally separated mice. Nature Communications, 6(1), 7735.

Desbonnet, L., Clarke, G., Shanahan, F., Dinan, T. G., & Cryan, J. F. (2014). Microbiota is essential for social development in the mouse. *Molecular Psychiatry*, 19(2), 146–8.

Desbonnet, L., Garrett, L., Clarke, G., Bienenstock, J., & Dinan, T. G. (2008). The probiotic Bifidobacteria infantis: An assessment of potential antidepressant properties in the rat. *Journal of Psychiatric Research*, 43(2), 164–174.

Desbonnet, L., Garrett, L., Clarke, G., Kiely, B., Cryan, J. F., & Dinan, T. G. (2010). Effects of the probiotic Bifidobacterium infantis in the maternal separation model of depression. *Neuroscience*, 170(4), 1179–1188.

Dinan,T. G. et al. (2013) Psychobiotics: A Novel Class of Psychotropic. Biol Psychiatry 2013;74:720–726

Distrutti, E., O'Reilly, J. A., McDonald, C., Cipriani, S., Renga, B., Lynch, M. A., & Fiorucci, S. (2014). Modulation of intestinal microbiota by the probiotic VSL#3 resets brain gene expression and ameliorates the age-related deficit in LTP. *PLoS ONE*, 9(9), e106503.

Dominguez-Bello, M. G., Costello, E. K., Contreras, M., Magris, M., Hidalgo, G., Fierer, N., & Knight, R. (2010). Delivery mode shapes the acquisition and structure of the initial microbiota across multiple body habitats in newborns. *Proceedings of the National Academy of Sciences of the United States of America*, 107(26), 11971–5.

Ellsworth, P. C. (1994). William James and Emotion: Is a Century of Fame Worth a Century of Misunderstanding? *Psychological Review*, 101(2), 222–229.

Eskelinen, M. H., Ngandu, T., Tuomilehto, J., Soininen, H., & Kivipelto, M. (2009). Midlife Coffee and Tea Drinking and the Risk of Late-Life Dementia: A Population-Based CAIDE Study. *Journal of Alzheimer's Disease*, 16(1), 85–91.

Fakhoury, M. (2015). Autistic spectrum disorders: A review of clinical features, theories and diagnosis. *International Journal of Developmental Neuroscience*, 43, 70–77.

Finegold, S. M., Dowd, S. E., Gontcharova, V., Liu, C., Henley, K. E., Wolcott, R. D., ... Green, J. A. (2010). Pyrosequencing study of fecal microflora of autistic and control children. *Anaerobe*, 16(4), 444–453.

Fond, G., Loundou, A., Hamdani, N., Boukouaci, W., Dargel, A., Oliveira, J., ... Boyer, L. (2014). Anxiety and depression comorbidities in irritable bowel syndrome (IBS): a systematic review and meta-analysis. *European Archives of Psychiatry and Clinical Neuroscience*, 264(8), 651–660.

Forsyth, C. B., Shannon, K. M., Kordower, J. H., Voigt, R. M., Shaikh, M., Jaglin, J. A., ... Keshavarzian, A. (2011). Increased intestinal permeability correlates with sigmoid mucosa alpha-synuclein staining and endotoxin exposure markers in early Parkinson's disease. *PLoS ONE*, 6(12).

Frémont, M., Coomans, D., Massart, S., & De Meirleir, K. (2013). High-throughput 16S rRNA gene sequencing reveals alterations of intestinal microbiota in myalgic encephalomyelitis/chronic fatigue syndrome patients. *Anaerobe*, 22, 50–56.

Gallup. (2017). Eight in 10 Americans Afflicted by Stress. https://news.gallup.com/poll/224336/eight-americans-afflicted-stress.aspx.

Gianaros, P. J., Jennings, J. R., Sheu, L. K., Greer, P. J., Kuller, L. H., & Matthews, K. A. (2007). Prospective reports of chronic life stress predict decreased grey matter volume in the hippocampus. *NeuroImage*, 35(2), 795–803.

Global Health Data Exchange. (2016). Global Burden of Disease. http://ghdx.healthdata.org/gbd-results-tool (accessed March 28, 2018).

Gondalia, S. V., Palombo, E. A., Knowles, S. R., Cox, S. B., Meyer, D., & Austin, D. W. (2012). Molecular Characterisation of Gastrointestinal Microbiota of Children With Autism (With and Without Gastrointestinal Dysfunction) and Their Neurotypical Siblings. *Autism Research*, 5(6), 419–427.

Govindarajan, N., Agis-Balboa, R. C., Walter, J., Sananbenesi, F., & Fischer, A. (2011). Sodium butyrate improves memory function in an alzheimer's disease mouse model when administered at an advanced stage of disease progression. *Journal of Alzheimer's Disease*, 26(1), 187–197.

Guida, F., Turco, F., Iannotta, M., De Gregorio, D., Palumbo, I., Sarnelli, G., ... Maione, S. (2018). Antibiotic-induced microbiota perturbation causes gut endocannabinoidome changes, hippocampal neuroglial reorganization and depression in mice. *Brain, Behavior, and Immunity*, 67, 230–245.

Gustavsson, A., Svensson, M., Jacobi, F., Allgulander, C., Alonso, J., Beghi, E., ... CDBE2010Study Group. (2011). Cost of disorders of the brain in Europe 2010. *European Neuropsychopharmacology: The Journal of the European College of Neuropsychopharmacology*, 21(10), 718–79.

Ha, S., Sohn, I.-J., Kim, N., Sim, H. J., & Cheon, K.-A. (2015). Characteristics of Brains in Autism Spectrum Disorder: Structure, Function and Connectivity across the Lifespan. *Experimental Neurobiology*, 24(4), 273–84.

Hasegawa, S., Goto, S., Tsuji, H., Okuno, T., Asahara, T., Nomoto, K., ... Hirayama, M. (2015). Intestinal dysbiosis and lowered serum lipopolysaccharide-binding protein in Parkinson's disease. *PLoS ONE*, 10(11), 1–15.

Hebert, L. E., Weuve, J., Scherr, P. A., & Evans, D. A. (2013). Alzheimer disease in the United States (2010-2050) estimated using the 2010 census. *Neurology*, 80(19), 1778–83.

Hsiao, E. Y., Mcbride, S. W., Hsien, S., Sharon, G., Hyde, E. R., Mccue, T., ... Mazmanian, S. K. (2014). The microbiota modulates gut physiology and behavioural abnormalities associated with autism. *Cell*, 155(7), 1451–1463.

Iovene, M. R., Bombace, F., Maresca, R., Sapone, A., Iardino, P., Picardi, A., ... Bravaccio, C. (2017). Intestinal Dysbiosis and Yeast Isolation in Stool of Subjects with Autism Spectrum Disorders. *Mycopathologia*, 182(3–4), 349–363.

Jaquet, M., Rochat, I., Moulin, J., Cavin, C., & Bibiloni, R. (2009). Impact of coffee consumption on the gut microbiota: A human volunteer study. *International Journal of Food Microbiology*, 130(2), 117–121.

Jiang, H., Ling, Z., Zhang, Y., Mao, H., Ma, Z., Yin, Y., ... Ruan, B. (2015). Altered fecal microbiota composition in patients with major depressive disorder. *Brain, Behavior, and Immunity*, 48, 186–194.

Kalliomäki, M., Carmen Collado, M., Salminen, S., & Isolauri, E. (2008). Early differences in fecal microbiota composition in children may predict overweight. *American Journal of Clinical Nutrition*, 87(3), 534–538.

Kang, D.-W., Adams, J. B., Gregory, A. C., Borody, T., Chittick, L., Fasano, A., ... Krajmalnik-Brown, R. (2017). Microbiota Transfer Therapy alters gut ecosystem and improves gastrointestinal and autism symptoms: an open-label study. *Microbiome*, 5(1), 10.

Kang, D. W., Park, J. G., Ilhan, Z. E., Wallstrom, G., LaBaer, J., Adams, J. B., & Krajmalnik-Brown, R. (2013). Reduced Incidence of Prevotella and Other Fermenters in Intestinal Microflora of Autistic Children. *PLoS ONE*, 8(7).

Kantarcioglu, A. S., Kiraz, N., & Aydin, A. (2016). Microbiota–Gut–Brain Axis: Yeast Species Isolated from Stool Samples of Children with Suspected or Diagnosed Autism Spectrum Disorders and In Vitro Susceptibility Against Nystatin and Fluconazole. *Mycopathologia*, 181(1–2), 1–7.

Keshavarzian, A., Green, S. J., Engen, P. A., Voigt, R. M., Naqib, A., Forsyth, C. B., ... Shannon, K. M. (2015). Colonic bacterial composition in Parkinson's disease. *Movement Disorders*, 30(10), 1351–1360.

Knivsberg, A. M., Reichelt, K. L., HØien, T., & NØdland, M. (2002). A Randomised, Controlled Study of Dietary Intervention in Autistic Syndromes. *Nutritional Neuroscience*, 5(4), 251–261.

Krakowiak, P., Walker, C. K., Bremer, A. A., Baker, A. S., Ozonoff, S., Hansen, R. L., & Hertz-Picciotto, I. (2012). Maternal metabolic conditions and risk for autism and other neurodevelopmental disorders. *Pediatrics*, 129(5), e1121-8.



Lebouvier, T. et al. (2008). Pathological lesions in colon biopsies during Parkinson's disease. *Gut* 57: 1741–1743

Leclercq, S., Matamoros, S., Cani, P. D., Neyrinck, A. M., Jamar, F., Starkel, P., ... Delzenne, N. M. (2014). Intestinal permeability, gut-bacterial dysbiosis, and behavioral markers of alcohol-dependence severity. *Proceedings of the National Academy of Sciences of the United States of America*, 111(42), E4485-93.

Lee, M., McGeer, E. G., & McGeer, P. L. (2016). Quercetin, not caffeine, is a major neuroprotective component in coffee. *Neurobiology of Aging*, 46, 113–23.

Li, W., Wu, X., Hu, X., Wang, T., Liang, S., Duan, Y., ... Qin, B. (2017). Structural changes of gut microbiota in Parkinson's disease and its correlation with clinical features. *Science China Life Sciences*, 60(11), 1223–1233.

Liu, B., Liu, J., Wang, M., Zhang, Y., & Li, L. (2017). From Serotonin to Neuroplasticity: Evolvement of Theories for Major Depressive Disorder. *Frontiers in Cellular Neuroscience*, 11, 305.

Liu, W.-H., Chuang, H.-L., Huang, Y.-T., Wu, C.-C., Chou, G.-T., Wang, S., & Tsai, Y.-C. (2016). Alteration of behavior and monoamine levels attributable to Lactobacillus plantarum PS128 in germ-free mice. *Behavioural Brain Research*, 298, 202–209.

Luczynski, P., McVey Neufeld, K.-A., Oriach, C. S., Clarke, G., Dinan, T. G., & Cryan, J. F. (2016). Growing up in a Bubble: Using Germ-Free Animals to Assess the Influence of the Gut Microbiota on Brain and Behavior. *International Journal of Neuropsychopharmacology*, 19(8), pyw020.

Luczynski, P., Whelan, S. O., O'Sullivan, C., Clarke, G., Shanahan, F., Dinan, T. G., & Cryan, J. F. (2016). Adult microbiota-deficient mice have distinct dendritic morphological changes: differential effects in the amygdala and hippocampus. *European Journal of Neuroscience*, 44(9), 2654–2666.

Macedo, D., Filho, A. J. M. C., Soares de Sousa, C. N., Quevedo, J., Barichello, T., Júnior, H. V. N., & Freitas de Lucena, D. (2017). Antidepressants, antimicrobials or both? Gut microbiota dysbiosis in depression and possible implications of the antimicrobial effects of antidepressant drugs for antidepressant effectiveness. *Journal of Affective Disorders*, 208, 22–32.

Maes, M., Kubera, M., & Leunis, J.-C. (2008). The gut-brain barrier in major depression: intestinal mucosal dysfunction with an increased translocation of LPS from gram negative enterobacteria (leaky gut) plays a role in the inflammatory pathophysiology of depression. *Neuro Endocrinology Letters*, 29(1), 117–24.

Mankad, D., Dupuis, A., Smile, S., Roberts, W., Brian, J., Lui, T., ... Anagnostou, E. (2015). A randomized, placebo controlled trial of omega-3 fatty acids in the treatment of young children with autism. *Molecular Autism*, 6(1), 18.

Martín, R., Langa, S., Reviriego, C., Jimínez, E., Marín, M. L., Xaus, J., ... Rodríguez, J. M. (2003). Human milk is a source of lactic acid bacteria for the infant gut. *Journal of Pediatrics*, 143(6), 754–8.

Martinez, J. M., Garakani, A., Yehuda, R., & Gorman, J. M. (2012). Proinflammatory and »resiliency« proteins in the CSF of patients with major depression. *Depression and Anxiety*, 29(1), 32–38.

Mathers, C. D., & Loncar, D. (2006). Projections of global mortality and burden of disease from 2002 to 2030. *PLoS Medicine*, 3(11), 2011–2030.

Mayer, E. A., Padua, D., & Tillisch, K. (2014). Altered brain-gut axis in autism: Comorbidity or causative mechanisms? *BioEssays*, 36(10), 933–939.

McKeown, C., Hisle-Gorman, E., Eide, M., Gorman, G. H., & Nylund, C. M. (2013). Association of constipation and fecal incontinence with attention-deficit/hyperactivity disorder. *Pediatrics*, 132(5), e1210-5.

Messaoudi, M., Lalonde, R., Violle, N., Javelot, H., Desor, D., Nejdi, A., ... Cazaubiel, J.-M. (2011). Assessment of psychotropic-like properties of a probiotic formulation (Lactobacillus helveticus R0052 and Bifidobacterium longum R0175) in rats and human subjects. *British Journal of Nutrition*, 105(5), 755–764.

Millward, C., Ferriter, M., Calver, S. J., & Connell-Jones, G. G. (2008). Gluten- and casein-free diets for autistic spectrum disorder. Cochrane Database of Systematic Reviews.

Minter, M. R., Zhang, C., Leone, V., Ringus, D. L., Zhang, X., Oyler-Castrillo, P., ... Sisodia, S. S. (2016). Antibiotic-induced perturbations in gut microbial diversity influences neuro-inflammation and amyloidosis in a murine model of Alzheimer's disease. *Sci Rep*, 6(July), 30028.

Miyauchi, E., Morita, H., & Tanabe, S. (2009). Lactobacillus rhamnosus alleviates intestinal barrier dysfunction in part by increasing expression of zonula occludens-1 and myosin light-chain kinase in vivo. *Journal of Dairy Science*, 92(6), 2400–8.

Mohd, R. S. (2008). Life Event, Stress and Illness, *Malaysian Journal of Medical Sciences*, 15(4), 9–18. https://www.ncbi.nlm.nih.gov/pmc/articles/PMC3341916/.

Möhle, L., Mattei, D., Heimesaat, M. M., Bereswill, S., Fischer, A., Alutis, M., ... Wolf, S. A. (2016). Ly6Chi Monocytes Provide a Link between Antibiotic-Induced Changes in Gut Microbiota and Adult Hippocampal Neurogenesis. *Cell Reports*, 15(9), 1945–1956.

Naseribafrouei, A., Hestad, K., Avershina, E., Sekelja, M., Linløkken, A., Wilson, R., & Rudi, K. (2014). Correlation between the human fecal microbiota and depression. *Neurogastroenterology and Motility*, 26(8), 1155–1162.

OECD. (2013). *Mental Health and Work: Sweden*. OECD Publishing.

Ogbonnaya, E. S., Clarke, G., Shanahan, F., Dinan, T. G., Cryan, J. F., & O'Leary, O. F. (2015). Adult Hippocampal Neurogenesis Is Regulated by the Microbiome. *Biological Psychiatry*, 78(4), e7–e9.

Ooi, Y. P., Weng, S.-J., Jang, L. Y., Low, L., Seah, J., Teo, S., ... Sung, M. (2015). Omega-3 fatty acids in the management of autism spectrum disorders: findings from an open-label pilot study in Singapore. European *Journal of Clinical Nutrition*, 69(8), 969–971.

Painsipp, E., Köfer, M. J., Sinner, F., & Holzer, P. (2011). Prolonged Depression-Like Behavior Caused by Immune Challenge: Influence of Mouse Strain and Social Environment. *PLoS ONE*, 6(6), e20719.

Parens, E., & Johnston, J. (2009). Facts, values, and Attention-Deficit Hyperactivity Disorder (ADHD): an update on the controversies. *Child and Adolescent Psychiatry and Mental Health*, 3(1), 1.

Parkinson Förbundet. (2014). Vad är Parkinson. http://www.parkinsonforbundet.se/index.html?id=2144 (accessed March 29, 2018).

Parkinson's Foundation. Statistics. https://parkinson.org/Understanding-Parkinsons/Statistics.

Parracho, H. M. R. T., Bingham, M. O., Gibson, G. R., & McCartney, A. L. (2005). Differences between the gut microflora of children with autistic spectrum disorders and that of healthy children. *Journal of Medical Microbiology*, 54(10), 987–991.

Pennesi, C. M., & Klein, L. C. (2012). Effectiveness of the gluten-free, casein-free diet for children diagnosed with autism spectrum disorder: Based on parental report. *Nutritional Neuroscience*, 15(2), 85–91.

Petrov, V. A., Saltykova, I. V., Zhukova, I. A., Alifirova, V. M., Zhukova, N. G., Dorofeeva, Y. B., ... Sazonov, A. E. (2017). Analysis of Gut Microbiota in Patients with Parkinson's Disease. *Bulletin of Experimental Biology and Medicine*, 162(6), 734–737.

Pinto-Sanchez, M. I., Hall, G. B., Ghajar, K., Nardelli, A., Bolino, C., Lau, J. T., ... Bercik, P. (2017). Probiotic Bifidobacterium longum NCC3001 Reduces Depression Scores and Alters Brain Activity: A Pilot Study in Patients With Irritable Bowel Syndrome. *Gastroenterology*, 77(0), 1282–1289.

Polanczyk, G., Silva de Lima, M., Lessa Horta, B., Biederman, J., & Augusto Rohde, L. (2007). The Worldwide Prevalence of ADHD: A Systematic Review and Metaregression Analysis. *Am J Psychiatry*, 1646.

Poole, R., Kennedy, O. J., Roderick, P., Fallowfield, J. A., Hayes, P. C., & Parkes, J. (2017). Coffee consumption and health: umbrella review of meta-analyses of multiple health outcomes. *BMJ*, 359, j5024.

Prince, M., Ali, G.-C., Guerchet, M., Prina, A. M., Albanese, E., & Wu, Y.-T. (2016). Recent global trends in the prevalence and incidence of dementia, and survival with dementia. *Alzheimer's Research {&} Therapy*, 8(1), 23.



Pärtty, A., Kalliomäki, M., Wacklin, P., Salminen, S., & Isolauri, E. (2015). A possible link between early probiotic intervention and the risk of neuropsychiatric disorders later in childhood - a randomized trial. *Pediatric Research*, 77(6), 823–828.

Qin, J., Li, R., Raes, J., Arumugam, M., Burgdorf, K. S., Manichanh, C., ... Wang, J. (2010). A human gut microbial gene catalogue established by metagenomic sequencing. *Nature*, 464(7285), 59–65.

Ravnkilde, B. (2004). Hippocampal volume and depression: a meta-analysis of MRI studies. *American Journal of Psychiatry*, 161(11), 1957–1966.

Reolon, G. K., Maurmann, N., Werenicz, A., Garcia, V. A., Schröder, N., Wood, M. A., & Roesler, R. (2011). Posttraining systemic administration of the histone deacetylase inhibitor sodium butyrate ameliorates aging-related memory decline in rats. *Behavioural Brain Research*, 221(1), 329–332.

Réus, G. Z., Fries, G. R., Stertz, L., Badawy, M., Passos, I. C., Barichello, T., ... Quevedo, J. (2015). The role of inflammation and microglial activation in the pathophysiology of psychiatric disorders. *Neuroscience*, 300, 141–154.

Ruskin, D. N., Svedova, J., Cote, J. L., Sandau, U., Rho, J. M., Kawamura, M., ... Masino, S. A. (2013). Ketogenic Diet Improves Core Symptoms of Autism in BTBR Mice. *PLoS ONE*, 8(6), e65021.

Sampson, T. R., Debelius, J. W., Thron, T., Janssen, S., Shastri, G. G., Ilhan, Z. E., ... Mazmanian, S. K. (2016). Gut Microbiota Regulate Motor Deficits and Neuroinflammation in a Model of Parkinson's Disease. *Cell*, 167(6), 1469–1480.e12.

Sandler, R. H., Finegold, S. M., Bolte, E. R., Buchanan, C. P., Maxwell, A. P., Väisänen, M.-L., ... Wexler, H. M. (2000). Short-Term Benefit From Oral Vancomycin Treatment of Regressive-Onset Autism. *Journal of Child Neurology*, 15(7), 429–435.

Santarelli, L., Saxe, M., Gross, C., Surget, A., Battaglia, F., Dulawa, S., ... Hen, R. (2003). Requirement of hippocampal neurogenesis for the behavioral effects of antidepressants. *Science* (New York, N.Y.), 301(5634), 805–9.

Saulnier, D. M., Riehle, K., Mistretta, T.-A., Diaz, M.-A., Mandal, D., Raza, S., ... Versalovic, J. (2011). Gastrointestinal microbiome signatures of pediatric patients with irritable bowel syndrome. *Gastroenterology*, 141(5), 1782–91.

Scheperjans, F., Aho, V., Pereira, P. A. B., Koskinen, K., Paulin, L., Pekkonen, E., ... Auvinen, P. (2015). Gut microbiota are related to Parkinson's disease and clinical phenotype. *Movement Disorders*, 30(3), 350–358.

Schmidt, K., Cowen, P. J., Harmer, C. J., Tzortzis, G., Errington, S., & Burnet, P. W. J. (2015). Prebiotic intake reduces the waking cortisol response and alters emotional bias in healthy volunteers. *Psychopharmacology*, 232(10), 1793–1801.

Schultz, S. T., Klonoff-Cohen, H. S., Wingard, D. L., Akshoomoff, N. A., Macera, C. A., Ji, M., & Bacher, C. (2006). Breastfeeding, infant formula supplementation, and Autistic Disorder: the results of a parent survey. *International Breastfeeding Journal*, 1(1), 16.

Shaaban, S. Y., Gendy, Y. G. El, Mehanna, N. S., El-Senousy, W. M., El-Feki, H. S. A., Saad, K., & El-Asheer, O. M. (2017). The role of probiotics in children with autism spectrum disorder: A prospective, open-label study. *Nutritional Neuroscience*, 0(0), 1–6.

Sharma, S., & Fulton, S. (2013). Diet-induced obesity promotes depressive-like behaviour that is associated with neural adaptations in brain reward circuitry. *International Journal of Obesity*, 37(3), 382–389.

Socialstyrelsen. (2016). Statistikdatabas för dödsorsaker. http://www.socialstyrelsen.se/statistik/statistikdatabas/dodsorsaker (accessed March 28, 2018).

Socialstyrelsen. (2017). Tillståndet och utvecklingen inom hälso- och sjukvård - Lägesrapport 2017. http://www.socialstyrelsen.se/Lists/Artikelkatalog/Attachments/20470/2017-3-1.pdf.

Spencer, S. J., Korosi, A., Layé, S., Shukitt-Hale, B., & Barrientos, R. M. (2017). Food for thought: how nutrition impacts cognition and emotion. *Science of Food*, 1(1), 7.

Steenbergen, L., Sellaro, R., van Hemert, S., Bosch, J. A., & Colzato, L. S. (2015). A randomized controlled trial to test the effect of multispecies probiotics on cognitive reactivity to sad mood. *Brain, Behavior, and Immunity*, 48, 258–264.

Strati, F., Cavalieri, D., Albanese, D., De Felice, C., Donati, C., Hayek, J., ... De Filippo, C. (2017). New evidences on the altered gut microbiota in autism spectrum disorders. *Microbiome*, 5(1), 24.

Sudo, N., Chida, Y., Aiba, Y., Sonoda, J., Oyama, N., Yu, X. N., ... Koga, Y. (2004). Postnatal microbial colonization programs the hypothalamic-pituitary-adrenal system for stress response in mice. *Journal of Physiology*, 558(1), 263–275.

The 1st International Conference on Microbiota-Gut-Brain Axis - Scientific Report. (2016). https://www.bastiaanse-communication.com/MMM2016/media/Scientific Report.pdf.

Thompson, R. S., Roller, R., Mika, A., Greenwood, B. N., Knight, R., Chichlowski, M., ... Fleshner, M. (2017). Dietary Prebiotics and Bioactive Milk Fractions Improve NREM Sleep, Enhance REM Sleep Rebound and Attenuate the Stress-Induced Decrease in Diurnal Temperature and Gut Microbial Alpha Diversity. *Frontiers in Behavioral Neuroscience*, 10(January), 240.

Tillisch Kirsten, L. J. et al. (2014). Consumption of Fermented Milk Product with Probiotics Modulates Brain Activity. *Gastroenterology*, 144(7), 1–15.

Unger, M. M., Spiegel, J., Dillmann, K.-U., Grundmann, D., Philippeit, H., Bürmann, J., ... Schäfer, K.-H. (2016). Short chain fatty acids and gut microbiota differ between patients with Parkinson's disease and age-matched controls. *Parkinsonism & Related Disorders*, 32, 66–72.

Vanuytsel, T., van Wanrooy, S., Vanheel, H., Vanormelingen, C., Verschueren, S., Houben, E., ... Tack, J. (2014). Psychological stress and corticotropin-releasing hormone increase intestinal permeability in humans by a mast cell-dependent mechanism. *Gut*, 63(8), 1293–9.

Visser, J., & Jehan, Z. (2009). ADHD: a scientific fact or a factual opinion? A critique of the veracity of Attention Deficit Hyperactivity Disorder. *Emotional and Behavioural Difficulties*, 14(2), 127–140.

Vlisidou, I., Lyte, M., van Diemen, P. M., Hawes, P., Monaghan, P., Wallis, T. S., & Stevens, M. P. (2004). The neuroendocrine stress hormone norepinephrine augments Escherichia coli O157:H7-induced enteritis and adherence in a bovine ligated ileal loop model of infection. *Infection and Immunity*, 72(9), 5446–51.

Vogelzangs, N., Duivis, H. E., Beekman, A. T. F., Kluft, C., Neuteboom, J., Hoogendijk, W., ... Penninx, B. W. J. H. (2012). Association of depressive disorders, depression characteristics and antidepressant medication with inflammation. *Translational Psychiatry*, 2(2), e79–e79.

Vogt, N. M., Kerby, R. L., Dill-McFarland, K. A., Harding, S. J., Merluzzi, A. P., Johnson, S. C., ... Rey, F. E. (2017). Gut microbiome alterations in Alzheimer's disease. *Scientific Reports*, 7(1), 13537.

Vos, T., Allen, C., Arora, M., Barber, R. M., Brown, A., Carter, A., ... Zuhlke, L. J. (2016). Global, regional, and national incidence, prevalence, and years lived with disability for 310 diseases and injuries, 1990–2015: a systematic analysis for the Global Burden of Disease Study 2015. *The Lancet*, 388(10053), 1545–1602.

Walker, E. A., Katon, W. J., Jemelka, R. P., & Roy-Byrne, P. P. (1992). Comorbidity of gastrointestinal complaints, depression, and anxiety in the epidemiologic catchment area (ECA) study. *American Journal of Medicine*, 92(1), S26–S30.

Wallace, C., Milev, R. (2017) The effects of probiotics on depressive symptoms in humans: a systematic review. *Ann Gen Psychiatry* (2017) 16:14

West, D. R., Roberst, E., Sichel, L. S., & Sichel, J. (2013). Improvements in Gastrointestinal Symptoms among Children with Autism Spectrum Disorder Receiving the Delpro® Probiotic and Immunomodulator Formulation. *Probiotics & Health*, 1(1), 1–6.



Zijlmans, M. A. C., Korpela, K., Riksen-Walraven, J. M., de Vos, W. M., & de Weerth, C. (2015). Maternal prenatal stress is associated with the infant intestinal microbiota. *Psychoneuroendocrinology*, 53, 233–245.

## CHAPTER 4

Abrams, S. A., Hawthorne, K. M., Aliu, O., Hicks, P. D., Chen, Z., & Griffin, I. J. (2007). An Inulin-Type Fructan Enhances CalciumAbsorption Primarily via an Effect on Colonic Absorption in Humans. *Journal of Nutrition*, 137(10), 2208–2212.

Adams, J. B., Romdalvik, J., Ramanujam, V. M. S., & Legator, M. S. (2007). Mercury, Lead, and Zinc in Baby Teeth of Children with Autism Versus Controls. *Journal of Toxicology and Environmental Health, Part A*, 70(12), 1046–1051.

Allen, A. P., Hutch, W., Borre, Y. E., Kennedy, P. J., Temko, A., Boylan, G., ... Clarke, G. (2016). Bifidobacterium longum 1714 as a translational psychobiotic: modulation of stress, electrophysiology and neurocognition in healthy volunteers. *Translational Psychiatry*, 6(11), e939.

American Heart Association. (2015). What is Metabolic Syndrome? https://www.heart.org/-/media/data-import/downloadables/pe-abh-what-is-metabolic-syndrome-ucm_300322.pdf.

American Psychological Association. (2017). Stress in America: Coping with Change. https://www.apa.org/news/press/releases/stress/2016/coping-with-change.pdf.

Anderson, S. C., Cryan, J. F. (John F. ., & Dinan, T. G. (2017). *The Psychobiotic Revolution: Mood, Food, and the New Science of the Gut-Brain Connection*. Washington: National Geographic Partners.

Aune, D., Chan, D. S. M., Lau, R., Vieira, R., Greenwood, D. C., Kampman, E., & Norat, T. (2011). Dietary fibre, whole grains, and risk of colorectal cancer: systematic review and dose-response meta-analysis of prospective studies. *BMJ* (Clinical research ed.), 343, d6617.

Barton, W., Penney, N. C., Cronin, O., Garcia-Perez, I., Molloy, M. G., Holmes, E., ... O'Sullivan, O. (2018). The microbiome of professional athletes differs from that of more sedentary subjects in composition and particularly at the functional metabolic level. *Gut*, 67(4), 625–633.

Benton, D., Williams, C., & Brown, A. (2007). Impact of consuming a milk drink containing a probiotic on mood and cognition. *European Journal of Clinical Nutrition*, 61(3), 355–361.

Bercik, P., Denou, E., Collins, J., Jackson, W., Lu, J., Jury, J., ... Collins, S. M. (2011). The Intestinal Microbiota Affect Central Levels of Brain-Derived Neurotropic Factor and Behavior in Mice. *Gastroenterology*, 141(2), 599–609.e3.

Bercik, P., Verdu, E. F., Foster, J. A., MacRi, J., Potter, M., Huang, X., ... Collins, S. M. (2010). Chronic gastrointestinal inflammation induces anxiety-like behavior and alters central nervous system biochemistry in mice. *Gastroenterology*, 139(6), 2102–2112.

Bergheim, I., Weber, S., Vos, M., Krämer, S., Volynets, V., Kaserouni, S., ... Bischoff, S. C. (2008). Antibiotics protect against fructose-induced hepatic lipid accumulation in mice: role of endotoxin. *Journal of Hepatology*, 48(6), 983–92.

Bravo, J. A., Forsythe, P., Chew, M. V, Escaravage, E., Savignac, H. M., Dinan, T. G., ... Cryan, J. F. (2011). Ingestion of Lactobacillus strain regulates emotional behavior and central GABA receptor expression in a mouse via the vagus nerve. *Proceedings of the National Academy of Sciences of the United States of America*, 108(38), 16050–5.

Buffington, S. A., Di Prisco, G. V., Auchtung, T. A., Ajami, N. J., Petrosino, J. F., & Costa-Mattioli, M. (2016). Microbial Reconstitution Reverses Maternal Diet-Induced Social and Synaptic Deficits in Offspring. *Cell*, 165(7), 1762–1775.

Burokas, A., Arboleya, S., Moloney, R. D., Peterson, V. L., Murphy, K., Clarke, G., ... Cryan, J. F. (2017). Targeting the Microbiota-Gut-Brain Axis: Prebiotics Have Anxiolytic and Antidepressant-like Effects and Reverse the Impact of Chronic Stress in Mice. *Biological Psychiatry*, 82(7), 472–487.

Cain, M. S., Leonard, J. A., Gabrieli, J. D. E., & Finn, A. S. (2016). Media multitasking in adolescence. *Psychonomic Bulletin & Review*, 23(6), 1932–1941.

Campana, R., Federici, S., Ciandrini, E., & Baffone, W. (2012). Antagonistic Activity of Lactobacillus acidophilus ATCC 4356 on the Growth and Adhesion/Invasion Characteristics of Human Campylobacter jejuni. *Current Microbiology*, 64(4), 371–378.

Canani, R. B., Costanzo, M. Di, Leone, L., Pedata, M., Meli, R., & Calignano, A. (2011). Potential beneficial effects of butyrate in intestinal and extraintestinal diseases. *World Journal of Gastroenterology*, 17(12), 1519–28.

Centers for Disease Control and Prevention. (2017). Antibiotic Use in the United States, 2017: Progress and Opportunities. https://www.cdc.gov/antibiotic-use/stewardship-report/outpatient.html (accessed April 2, 2018).

Centers for Disease Control and Prevention. (2017). Heart Disease Facts. https://www.cdc.gov/heartdisease/facts.htm.

Centers for Disease Control and Prevention. (2015). Nearly half a million Americans suffered from Clostridium difficile infections in a single year. https://www.cdc.gov/media/releases/2015/p0225-clostridium-difficile.html.

Chassaing, B., Koren, O., Goodrich, J. K., Poole, A. C., Srinivasan, S., Ley, R. E., & Gewirtz, A. T. (2015). Dietary emulsifiers impact the mouse gut microbiota promoting colitis and metabolic syndrome. *Nature*, 519(7541), 92–96.

Christ, A., Günther, P., Lauterbach, M. A. R., Duewell, P., Biswas, D., Pelka, K., ... Latz, E. (2018). Western Diet Triggers NLRP3-Dependent Innate Immune Reprogramming. *Cell*, 172(1–2), 162–175.e14.

Clemente, J. C., Pehrsson, E. C., Blaser, M. J., Sandhu, K., Gao, Z., Wang, B., ... Dominguez-Bello, M. G. (2015). The microbiome of uncontacted Amerindians. *Science Advances*, 1(3), e1500183–e1500183.

Daley, C. A., Abbott, A., Doyle, P. S., Nader, G. A., & Larson, S. (2010). A review of fatty acid profiles and antioxidant content in grass-fed and grain-fed beef. *Nutrition Journal*, 9, 10.

De Filippo, C., Cavalieri, D., Di Paola, M., Ramazzotti, M., Poullet, J. B., Massart, S., ... Lionetti, P. (2010). Impact of diet in shaping gut microbiota revealed by a comparative study in children from Europe and rural Africa. *Proceedings of the National Academy of Sciences of the United States of America*, 107(33), 14691–6.

De Palma, G., Lynch, M. D. J., Lu, J., Dang, V. T., Deng, Y., Jury, J., ... Bercik, P. (2017). Transplantation of fecal microbiota from patients with irritable bowel syndrome alters gut function and behavior in recipient mice. *Science Translational Medicine*, 9(379), eaaf6397.

Dewanto, V., Wu, X., Adom, K. K., & Liu, R. H. (2002). Thermal processing enhances the nutritional value of tomatoes by increasing total antioxidant activity. *Journal of Agricultural and Food Chemistry*, 50(10), 3010–4.

DiRienzo, D. B. (2014). Effect of probiotics on biomarkers of cardiovascular disease: implications for heart-healthy diets. *Nutrition Reviews*, 72(1), 18–29.

Durrer, K. E., Allen, M. S., & Hunt von Herbing, I. (2017). Genetically engineered probiotic for the treatment of phenylketonuria (PKU); assessment of a novel treatment in vitro and in the PAHenu2 mouse model of PKU. *PLOS ONE*, 12(5), e0176286.

van den Eijnden, R. J. J. M., Lemmens, J. S., & Valkenburg, P. M. (2016). The Social Media Disorder Scale. *Computers in Human Behavior*, 61, 478–487.

Erdman, S. E., & Poutahidis, T. (2014). Probiotic "glow of health": it's more than skin deep. *Beneficial Microbes*, 5(2), 109–119.

Estroff Marano, H. (2001). Depression Doing the Thinking. *Psychology Today*. https://www.psychologytoday.com/us/articles/200107/depression-doing-the-thinking.

Finnegan, M. (2015, juli). Faecal transplants may help treat clinical depression. *Irish Times*. https://www.irishtimes.com/news/science/faecal-transplants-may-help-treat-clinical-depression-1.2281161.

Foley, J. O., & DuBois, F. S. (1937). Quantitative studies of the vagus nerve in the cat. I. The ratio of sensory to motor fibers. *Journal of Comparative Neurology*, 67(1), 49–67.

Fåk, F., & Bäckhed, F. (2012). Lactobacillus reuteri Prevents Diet-Induced Obesity, but not Atherosclerosis, in a Strain Dependent Fashion in Apoe−/− Mice. *PLoS ONE*, 7(10), e46837.

Gargari, B. P., Namazi, N., Khalili, M., Sarmadi, B., Jafarabadi, M. A., & Dehghan, P. (2015). Is there any place for resistant starch, as alimentary prebiotic, for patients with type 2 diabetes? *Complementary Therapies in Medicine*, 23(6), 810–815.

Gautam, M., Agrawal, M., Gautam, M., Sharma, P., Gautam, A. S., & Gautam, S. (2012). Role of antioxidants in generalised anxiety disorder and depression. *Indian Journal of Psychiatry*, 54(3), 244–7.

Goldin, P., Ziv, M., Jazaieri, H., Hahn, K., & Gross, J. J. (2013). MBSR vs aerobic exercise in social anxiety: fMRI of emotion regulation of negative self-beliefs. *Social Cognitive and Affective Neuroscience*, 8(1), 65–72.

Goodrich, J. K., Waters, J. L., Poole, A. C., Sutter, J. L., Koren, O., Blekhman, R., ... Ley, R. E. (2014). Human genetics shape the gut microbiome. *Cell*, 159(4), 789–99.

Govindarajan, N., Agis-Balboa, R. C., Walter, J., Sananbenesi, F., & Fischer, A. (2011). Sodium butyrate improves memory function in an alzheimer's disease mouse model when administered at an advanced stage of disease progression. *Journal of Alzheimer's Disease*, 26(1), 187–197.

Green, A., Cohen-Zion, M., Haim, A., & Dagan, Y. (2017). Evening light exposure to computer screens disrupts human sleep, biological rhythms, and attention abilities. *Chronobiology International*, 34(7), 855–865.

Haahr, T., Glavind, J., Axelsson, P., Bistrup Fischer, M., Bjurström, J., Andrésdóttir, G., ... Clausen, T. (2017). Vaginal seeding or vaginal microbial transfer from the mother to the caesarean-born neonate: a commentary regarding clinical management. *BJOG: An International Journal of Obstetrics & Gynaecology*, 125(5), 533–536.

Harari, Y. N. (2014). *Sapiens: A Brief History of Mankind*. New York: Harper.

Hargrave, S. L., Davidson, T. L., Zheng, W., & Kinzig, K. P. (2016). Western diets induce blood-brain barrier leakage and alter spatial strategies in rats. *Behavioral Neuroscience*, 130(1), 123–135.

Hilimire, M. R., DeVylder, J. E., & Forestell, C. A. (2015). Fermented foods, neuroticism, and social anxiety: An interaction model. *Psychiatry Research*, 228(2), 203–208.

Hofmann, W., Vohs, K. D., & Baumeister, R. F. (2012). What People Desire, Feel Conflicted About, and Try to Resist in Everyday Life. *Psychological Science*, 23(6), 582–588.

Hsiao, E. Y., Mcbride, S. W., Hsien, S., Sharon, G., Hyde, E. R., Mccue, T., ... Mazmanian, S. K. (2014). The microbiota modulates gut physiology and behavioural abnormalities associated with autism. *Cell*, 155(7), 1451–1463.

Hsu, Y. J., Chiu, C. C., Li, Y. P., Huang, W. C., Huang, Y. Te, Huang, C. C., & Chuang, H. L. (2015). Effect of intestinal microbiota on exercise performance in mice. *Journal of Strength and Conditioning Research*, 29(2), 552–8.

Hu, Y., Long, X., Lyu, H., Zhou, Y., & Chen, J. (2017). Alterations in White Matter Integrity in Young Adults with Smartphone Dependence. *Frontiers in Human Neuroscience*, 11.

Jacka, F. N., Mykletun, A., Berk, M., Bjelland, I., & Tell, G. S. (2011). The Association Between Habitual Diet Quality and the Common Mental Disorders in Community-dwelling Adults: The Hordaland Health Study. *Psychosomatic Medicine*, 73(6), 483–490.

Jalanka, J., Hillamaa, A., Satokari, R., Mattila, E., Anttila, V.-J., & Arkkila, P. (2018). The long-term effects of faecal microbiota transplantation for gastrointestinal symptoms and general health in patients with recurrent Clostridium difficile infection. *Alimentary Pharmacology & Therapeutics*, 47(3), 371–379.

Jeong, J. J., Woo, J. Y., Kim, K. A., Han, M. J., & Kim, D. H. (2015). Lactobacillus pentosus var. plantarum C29 ameliorates age-dependent memory impairment in Fischer 344 rats. *Letters in Applied Microbiology*, 60(4), 307–314.

Jost, T., Lacroix, C., Braegger, C., & Chassard, C. (2015). Impact of human milk bacteria and oligosaccharides on neonatal gut microbiota establishment and gut health. *Nutrition Reviews*, 73(7), 426–437.

Kamiya, T., Wang, L., Forsythe, P., Goettsche, G., Mao, Y., Wang, Y., ... Bienenstock, J. (2006). Inhibitory effects of Lactobacillus reuteri on visceral pain induced by colorectal distension in Sprague-Dawley rats. *Gut*, 55(2), 191–6.

Kang, D.-W., Adams, J. B., Gregory, A. C., Borody, T., Chittick, L., Fasano, A., ... Krajmalnik-Brown, R. (2017). Microbiota Transfer Therapy alters gut ecosystem and improves gastrointestinal and autism symptoms: an open-label study. *Microbiome*, 5(1), 10.

Kelly, J. R., Borre, Y., O' Brien, C., Patterson, E., El Aidy, S., Deane, J., ... Dinan, T. G. (2016). Transferring the blues: Depression-associated gut microbiota induces neurobehavioural changes in the rat. *Journal of Psychiatric Research*, 82, 109–118.

Komatszaki, N., & Shima, J. (2012). Effects of Live *Lactobacillus paracasei* on Plasma Lipid Concentration in Rats Fed an Ethanol-Containing Diet. *Bioscience, Biotechnology, and Biochemistry*, 76(2), 232–237.

Kootte, R. S., Levin, E., Salojärvi, J., Smits, L. P., Hartstra, A. V., Udayappan, S. D., ... Nieuwdorp, M. (2017). Improvement of Insulin Sensitivity after Lean Donor Feces in Metabolic Syndrome Is Driven by Baseline Intestinal Microbiota Composition. *Cell Metabolism*, 26(4), 611–619.e6.

Kuo, S.-M. (2013). The Interplay Between Fiber and the Intestinal Microbiome in the Inflammatory Response. *Advances in Nutrition*, 4(1), 16–28.

Kuss, D. J., & Griffiths, M. D. (2011). Online Social Networking and Addiction—A Review of the Psychological Literature. *International Journal of Environmental Research and Public Health*, 8(9), 3528–3552.

Laugerette, F., Furet, J.-P., Debard, C., Daira, P., Loizon, E., Géloën, A., ... Michalski, M.-C. (2012). Oil composition of high-fat diet affects metabolic inflammation differently in connection with endotoxin receptors in mice. *American Journal of Physiology-Endocrinology and Metabolism*, 302(3), E374–E386.

Lazar, S. W., Kerr, C. E., Wasserman, R. H., Gray, J. R., Greve, D. N., Treadway, M. T., ... Fischl, B. (2005). Meditation experience is associated with increased cortical thickness. *Neuroreport*, 16(17), 1893–7.

Levenson, J. C., Shensa, A., Sidani, J. E., Colditz, J. B., & Primack, B. A. (2016). The association between social media use and sleep disturbance among young adults. *Preventive Medicine*, 85, 36–41.

Lewis, S. J., & Heaton, K. W. (1997). Increasing butyrate concentration in the distal colon by accelerating intestinal transit. *Gut*, 41(2), 245–51.

Li, W., Dowd, S. E., Scurlock, B., Acosta-Martinez, V., & Lyte, M. (2009). Memory and learning behavior in mice is temporally associated with diet-induced alterations in gut bacteria. *Physiology & Behavior*, 96(4–5), 557–67.

Li, Y., Lv, M.-R., Wei, Y.-J., Sun, L., Zhang, J.-X., Zhang, H.-G., & Li, B. (2017). Dietary patterns and depression risk: A meta-analysis. *Psychiatry Research*, 253, 373–382.

Li, Y., Shimizu, T., Hosaka, A., Kaneko, N., Ohtsuka, Y., & Yamashiro, Y. (2004). Effects of bifidobacterium breve supplementation on intestinal flora of low birth weight infants. *Pediatrics International*, 46(5), 509–515.



Lin, L. yi, Sidani, J. E., Shensa, A., Radovic, A., Miller, E., Colditz, J. B., ... Primack, B. A. (2016). Association between social media use and depression among U.S. young adults. *Depression and Anxiety*, 33(4), 323–331.

Lodge, C., Tan, D., Lau, M., Dai, X., Tham, R., Lowe, A., ... Dharmage, S. (2015). Breastfeeding and asthma and allergies: a systematic review and meta-analysis. *Acta Paediatrica*, 104(467), 38–53.

Logan, A. C., & Katzman, M. (2005). Major depressive disorder: probiotics may be an adjuvant therapy. *Medical Hypotheses*, 64(3), 533–8.

Luo, J., Wang, T., Liang, S., Hu, X., Li, W., & Jin, F. (2014). Ingestion of Lactobacillus strain reduces anxiety and improves cognitive function in the hyperammonemia rat. *Science China Life Sciences*, 57(3), 327–335.

Maki, K. C., Pelkman, C. L., Finocchiaro, E. T., Kelley, K. M., Lawless, A. L., Schild, A. L., & Rains, T. M. (2012). Resistant Starch from High-Amylose Maize Increases Insulin Sensitivity in Overweight and Obese Men. *Journal of Nutrition*, 142(4), 717–723.

Maldonado-Gómez, M. X., Martínez, I., Bottacini, F., O'Callaghan, A., Ventura, M., van Sinderen, D., ... Walter, J. (2016). Stable Engraftment of Bifidobacterium longum AH1206 in the Human Gut Depends on Individualized Features of the Resident Microbiome. *Cell Host & Microbe*, 20(4), 515–526.

Martarelli, D., Verdenelli, M. C., Scuri, S., Cocchioni, M., Silvi, S., Cecchini, C., & Pompei, P. (2011). Effect of a Probiotic Intake on Oxidant and Antioxidant Parameters in Plasma of Athletes During Intense Exercise Training. *Current Microbiology*, 62(6), 1689–1696.

Mathipa, M. G., & Thantsha, M. S. (2015). Cocktails of probiotics pre-adapted to multiple stress factors are more robust under simulated gastrointestinal conditions than their parental counterparts and exhibit enhanced antagonistic capabilities against Escherichia coli and Staphylococcus aureus. *Gut Pathogens*, 7, 5.

Matsumoto, M., Inoue, R., Tsukahara, T., Ushida, K., Cciji, H., Matsubara, N., & Hara, H. (2008). Voluntary Running Exercise Alters Microbiota Composition and Increases n-Butyrate Concentration in the Rat Cecum. *Bioscience, Biotechnology, and Biochemistry*, 72(2), 572–576.

Minter, M. R., Zhang, C., Leone, V., Ringus, D. L., Zhang, X., Oyler-Castrillo, P., ... Sisodia, S. S. (2016). Antibiotic-induced perturbations in gut microbial diversity influences neuro-inflammation and amyloidosis in a murine model of Alzheimer's disease. *Sci Rep*, 6(July), 30028.

Moisala, M., Salmela, V., Hietajärvi, L., Salo, E., Carlson, S., Salonen, O., ... Alho, K. (2016). Media multitasking is associated with distractibility and increased prefrontal activity in adolescents and young adults. *NeuroImage*, 134, 113–121.

Mosley, M. (2017). *Clever Guts Diet: How to Revolutionise Your Body from the Inside Out*. London: Short Books Ltd.

Mueller, N. T., Bakacs, E., Combellick, J., Grigoryan, Z., & Dominguez-Bello, M. G. (2015). The infant microbiome development: mom matters. *Trends in Molecular Medicine*, 21(2), 109–117.

Möhle, L., Mattei, D., Heimesaat, M. M., Bereswill, S., Fischer, A., Alutis, M., ... Wolf, S. A. (2016). Ly6Chi Monocytes Provide a Link between Antibiotic-Induced Changes in Gut Microbiota and Adult Hippocampal Neurogenesis. *Cell Reports*, 15(9), 1945–1956.

Niedzielin, K., Kordecki, H., & Birkenfeld, B. (2001). A controlled, double-blind, randomized study on the efficacy of Lactobacillus plantarum 299V in patients with irritable bowel syndrome. *European Journal of Gastroenterology & Hepatology*, 13(10), 1143–7.

O'Sullivan, O., Cronin, O., Clarke, S. F., Murphy, E. F., Molloy, M. G., Shanahan, F., & Cotter, P. D. (2015). Exercise and the microbiota. *Gut Microbes*, 6(2), 131–136.

Ohland, C. L., Kish, L., Bell, H., Thiesen, A., Hotte, N., Pankiv, E., & Madsen, K. L. (2013). Effects of Lactobacillus helveticus on murine behavior are dependent on diet and genotype and correlate with alterations in the gut microbiome. *Psychoneuroendocrinology*, 38(9), 1738–1747.

Pan, A., Sun, Q., Bernstein, A. M., Schulze, M. B., Manson, J. E., Stampfer, M. J., ... Hu, F. B. (2012). Red meat consumption and mortality: results from 2 prospective cohort studies. *Archives of Internal Medicine*, 172(7), 555–63.

Pedersen, N., Andersen, N. N., Végh, Z., Jensen, L., Ankersen, D. V., Felding, M., ... Munkholm, P. (2014). Ehealth: low FODMAP diet vs Lactobacillus rhamnosus GG in irritable bowel syndrome. *World Journal of Gastroenterology*, 20(43), 16215–26.

Peres, J. (2014). Resistant Starch May Reduce Colon Cancer Risk From Red Meat. *JNCI: Journal of the National Cancer Institute*, 106(10).

Perez-Cornago, A., Sanchez-Villegas, A., Bes-Rastrollo, M., Gea, A., Molero, P., Lahortiga-Ramos, F., & Martínez-González, M. A. (2016). Intake of High-Fat Yogurt, but Not of Low-Fat Yogurt or Prebiotics, Is Related to Lower Risk of Depression in Women of the SUN Cohort Study. *Journal of Nutrition*, 146(9), 1731–1739.

Phua, T., Sng, M. K., Tan, E. H. P., Chee, D. S. L., Li, Y., Wee, J. W. K., ... Tan, N. S. (2017). Angiopoietin-like 4 Mediates Colonic Inflammation by Regulating Chemokine Transcript Stability via Tristetraprolin. *Scientific Reports*, 7, 44351.

Pitkala, K. H., Strandberg, T. E., Finne Soveri, U. H., Ouwehand, A. C., Poussa, T., & Salminen, S. (2007). Fermented cereal with specific bifidobacteria normalizes bowel movements in elderly nursing home residents. A randomized, controlled trial. *Journal of Nutrition, Health & Aging*, 11(4), 305–311.

Plovier, H., Everard, A., Druart, C., Depommier, C., Van Hul, M., Geurts, L., ... Cani, P. D. (2017). A purified membrane protein from Akkermansia muciniphila or the pasteurized bacterium improves metabolism in obese and diabetic mice. *Nature Medicine*, 23(1), 107–113.

Primack, B. A., Shensa, A., Escobar-Viera, C. G., Barrett, E. L., Sidani, J. E., Colditz, J. B., & James, A. E. (2017). Use of multiple social media platforms and symptoms of depression and anxiety: A nationally-representative study among U.S. young adults. *Computers in Human Behavior*, 69, 1–9.

Przybylski, A. K., & Weinstein, N. (2017). A Large-Scale Test of the Goldilocks Hypothesis: Quantifying the Relations Between Digital-Screen Use and the Mental Well-Being of Adolescents. *Psychological Science*, 28(2), 204–215.

Pusceddu, M. M., El Aidy, S., Crispie, F., O'Sullivan, O., Cotter, P., Stanton, C., ... Dinan, T. G. (2015). N-3 Polyunsaturated Fatty Acids (PUFAs) Reverse the Impact of Early-Life Stress on the Gut Microbiota. *PLOS ONE*, 10(10), e0139721.

Ramiah, K., van Reenen, C. A., & Dicks, L. M. T. (2008). Surface-bound proteins of Lactobacillus plantarum 423 that contribute to adhesion of Caco-2 cells and their role in competitive exclusion and displacement of Clostridium sporogenes and Enterococcus faecalis. *Research in Microbiology*, 159(6), 470–475.

Rao, A. V., Bested, A. C., Beaulne, T. M., Katzman, M. A., Iorio, C., Berardi, J. M., & Logan, A. C. (2009). A randomized, double-blind, placebo-controlled pilot study of a probiotic in emotional symptoms of chronic fatigue syndrome. *Gut Pathogens*, 1(1), 6.

Reigstad, C. S., Salmonson, C. E., Rainey, J. F., Szurszewski, J. H., Linden, D. R., Sonnenburg, J. L., ... Kashyap, P. C. (2015). Gut microbes promote colonic serotonin production through an effect of short-chain fatty acids on enterochromaffin cells. *FASEB Journal: Official Publication of the Federation of American Societies for Experimental Biology*, 29(4), 1395–403.

Reinecke, L., Aufenanger, S., Beutel, M. E., Dreier, M., Quiring, O., Stark, B., ... Müller, K. W. (2017). Digital Stress over the Life Span: The Effects of Communication Load and Internet Multitasking on Perceived Stress and Psychological Health Impairments in a German Probability Sample. *Media Psychology*, 20(1), 90–115.

Remely, M., Hippe, B., Geretschlaeger, I., Stegmayer, S., Hoefinger, I., & Haslberger, A. (2015). Increased gut microbiota diversity and abundance of Faecalibacterium prausnitzii and Akkermansia after fasting: a pilot study. *Wiener klinische Wochenschrift*, 127(9–10), 394–398.

Review on Antimicrobial Resistance. (2016). Tackling Drug-resistant infections globally: Final Report and Recommendations. https://doi.org/10.1016/j.jpha.2015.11.005

Rousseaux, C., Thuru, X., Gelot, A., Barnich, N., Neut, C., Dubuquoy, L., ... Desreumaux, P. (2007). Lactobacillus acidophilus modulates intestinal pain and induces opioid and cannabinoid receptors. *Nature Medicine*, 13(1), 35–37.

Saavedra, J. ., Bauman, N. ., Perman, J. ., Yolken, R. ., Saavedra, J. ., Bauman, N. ., & Oung, I. (1994). Feeding of Bifidobacterium bifidum and Streptococcus thermophilus to infants in hospital for prevention of diarrhoea and shedding of rotavirus. *The Lancet*, 344(8929), 1046–1049.

Savignac, H. M., Couch, Y., Stratford, M., Bannerman, D. M., Tzortzis, G., Anthony, D. C., & Burnet, P. W. J. (2016). Prebiotic administration normalizes lipopolysaccharide (LPS)-induced anxiety and cortical 5-HT2A receptor and IL1-?? levels in male mice. *Brain, Behavior, and Immunity*, 52, 120–131.

Savignac, H. M., Kiely, B., Dinan, T. G., & Cryan, J. F. (2014). Bifidobacteria exert strain-specific effects on stress-related behavior and physiology in BALB/c mice. *Neurogastroenterology and Motility*, 26(11), 1615–1627.

Schmidt, K., Cowen, P. J., Harmer, C. J., Tzortzis, G., Errington, S., & Burnet, P. W. J. (2015). Prebiotic intake reduces the waking cortisol response and alters emotional bias in healthy volunteers. *Psychopharmacology*, 232(10), 1793–1801.

Schnorr, S. L., Candela, M., Rampelli, S., Centanni, M., Consolandi, C., Basaglia, G., ... Crittenden, A. N. (2014). Gut microbiome of the Hadza hunter-gatherers. *Nat Commun*, 5, 3654.

Shakya, H. B., & Christakis, N. A. (2017). Association of Facebook Use With Compromised Well-Being: A Longitudinal Study. *American Journal of Epidemiology*.

Sherman, L. E., Payton, A. A., Hernandez, L. M., Greenfield, P. M., & Dapretto, M. (2016). The Power of the Like in Adolescence. *Psychological Science*, 27(7), 1027–1035.

Silk, D. B. A., Davis, A., Vulevic, J., Tzortzis, G., & Gibson, G. R. (2009). Clinical trial: The effects of a trans-galactooligosaccharide prebiotic on faecal microbiota and symptoms in irritable bowel syndrome. *Alimentary Pharmacology and Therapeutics*, 29(5), 508–518.

Slavin, J. (2013). Fiber and prebiotics: mechanisms and health benefits. Nutrients, 5(4), 1417–35.

Spector, T. D. (2016). *The Diet Myth: Why the Secret to Health and Weight Loss Is Already in Your Gut.* New York: The Overlook Press.

Steenbergen, L., Sellaro, R., van Hemert, S., Bosch, J. A., & Colzato, L. S. (2015). A randomized controlled trial to test the effect of multispecies probiotics on cognitive reactivity to sad mood. *Brain, Behavior, and Immunity*, 48, 258–264.

Sutherland, J., Miles, M., Hedderley, D., Li, J., Devoy, S., Sutton, K., & Lauren, D. (2009). In vitro effects of food extracts on selected probiotic and pathogenic bacteria. *International Journal of Food Sciences and Nutrition*, 60(8), 717–727.

Taverniti, V., & Guglielmetti, S. (2012). Health-Promoting Properties of *Lactobacillus helveticus. Frontiers in Microbiology*, 3, 392.

Temmerman, R., Scheirlinck, I., Huys, G., & Swings, J. (2003). Culture-independent analysis of probiotic products by denaturing gradient gel electrophoresis. *Applied and Environmental Microbiology*, 69(1), 220–6.

The algorithm diet | Weizmann Institute of Science. (n.d.). http://www.weizmann.ac.il/pages/home/algorithm-diet (accessed April 3, 2018).

Thompson, R. S., Roller, R., Mika, A., Greenwood, B. N., Knight, R., Chichlowski, M., … Fleshner, M. (2017). Dietary Prebiotics and Bioactive Milk Fractions Improve NREM Sleep, Enhance REM Sleep Rebound and Attenuate the Stress-Induced Decrease in Diurnal Temperature and Gut Microbial Alpha Diversity. *Frontiers in Behavioral Neuroscience*, 10(January), 240.

Uncapher, M. R., K. Thieu, M., & Wagner, A. D. (2016). Media multitasking and memory: Differences in working memory and long-term memory. *Psychonomic Bulletin & Review*, 23(2), 483–490.

Varian, B. J., Poutahidis, T., DiBenedictis, B. T., Levkovich, T., Ibrahim, Y., Didyk, E., … Erdman, S. E. (2017). Microbial lysate upregulates host oxytocin. *Brain, Behavior, and Immunity*, 61, 36–49.

Verdú, E. F., Bercik, P., Verma-Gandhu, M., Huang, X.-X., Blennerhassett, P., Jackson, W., … Collins, S. M. (2006). Specific probiotic therapy attenuates antibiotic induced visceral hypersensitivity in mice. *Gut*, 55(2), 182–90.

Wang, R., Yang, F., & Haigh, M. M. (2017). Let me take a selfie: Exploring the psychological effects of posting and viewing selfies and groupies on social media. *Telematics and Informatics*, 34(4), 274–283.

WebMD. (n.d.). INULIN: Uses, Side Effects, Interactions and Warnings. https://www.webmd.com/vitamins-supplements/ingredientmono-1048-INULIN.aspx (accessed April 2, 2018).

Weir, H. J., Yao, P., Huynh, F. K., Escoubas, C. C., Goncalves, R. L., Burkewitz, K., … Mair, W. B. (2017). Dietary Restriction and AMPK Increase Lifespan via Mitochondrial Network and Peroxisome Remodeling. *Cell Metabolism*, 26(6), 884–896.e5.

Wilmer, H. H., & Chein, J. M. (2016). Mobile technology habits: patterns of association among device usage, intertemporal preference, impulse control, and reward sensitivity. *Psychonomic Bulletin & Review*, 23(5), 1607–1614.

Yassour, M., Vatanen, T., Siljander, H., Hämäläinen, A.-M., Härkönen, T., Ryhänen, S. J., … Xavier, R. J. (2016). Natural history of the infant gut microbiome and impact of antibiotic treatment on bacterial strain diversity and stability. *Science Translational Medicine*, 8(343), 343ra81.

Yatsunenko, T., Rey, F. E., Manary, M. J., Trehan, I., Dominguez-Bello, M. G., Contreras, M., ... Gordon, J. I. (May 9, 2012). Human gut microbiome viewed across age and geography. *Nature*. Nature Publishing Group.

Zatorre, R. J., Fields, R. D., & Johansen-Berg, H. (2012). Plasticity in gray and white: neuroimaging changes in brain structure during learning. *Nature Neuroscience*, 15(4), 528–536.

Zhang, C., Li, S., Yang, L., Huang, P., Li, W., Wang, S., ... Zhao, L. (2013). Structural modulation of gut microbiota in life-long calorie-restricted mice. *Nature Communications*, 4, 2163.

Zhang, M., & Yang, X.-J. (2016). Effects of a high fat diet on intestinal microbiota and gastrointestinal diseases. *World Journal of Gastroenterology*, 22(40), 8905–8909.

## CHAPTER 5

Ahn, G., Moon, J. S., Shin, S., Min, W. K., Han, N. S., & Seo, J. (2015). A competitive quantitative polymerase chain reaction method for characterizing the population dynamics during kimchi fermentation. *Journal of Industrial Microbiology & Biotechnology*, 42(1), 49–55.

An, S.-Y., Lee, M. S., Jeon, J. Y., Ha, E. S., Kim, T. H., Yoon, J. Y., ... Lee, K.-W. (2013). Beneficial Effects of Fresh and Fermented Kimchi in Prediabetic Individuals. *Ann Nutr Metab*, 63, 111–119.

Battikh, H., Bakhrouf, A., & Ammar, E. (2012). Antimicrobial effect of Kombucha analogues. *LWT - Food Science and Technology*, 47(1), 71–77.

Bauer-Petrovska, B., & Petrushevska-Tozi, L. (2000). Mineral and water soluble vitamin content in the Kombucha drink. *International Journal of Food Science and Technology*, 35(2), 201–205.



Bhattacharya, D., Bhattacharya, S., Patra, M. M., Chakravorty, S., Sarkar, S., Chakraborty, W., ... Gachhui, R. (2016). Antibacterial Activity of Polyphenolic Fraction of Kombucha Against Enteric Bacterial Pathogens. *Current Microbiology*, 73(6), 885–896.

Bonfili, L., Cecarini, V., Berardi, S., Scarpona, S., Suchodolski, J. S., Nasuti, C., ... Eleuteri, A. M. (2017). Microbiota modulation counteracts Alzheimer's disease progression influencing neuronal proteolysis and gut hormones plasma levels. *Scientific Reports*, 7(1), 2426.

Chakravorty, S., Bhattacharya, S., Chatzinotas, A., Chakraborty, W., Bhattacharya, D., & Gachhui, R. (2016). Kombucha tea fermentation: Microbial and biochemical dynamics. *International Journal of Food Microbiology*, 220, 63–72.

Cheigh, C. I., Choi, H. J., Park, H., Kim, S. B., Kook, M. C., Kim, T. S., ... Pyun, Y. R. (2002). Influence of growth conditions on the production of a nisin-like bacteriocin by Lactococcus lactis subsp. lactis A164 isolated from kimchi. *Journal of Biotechnology*, 95(3), 225–235.

Cheigh, H., Park, K., Lee, C. Y., Cheigh, H.-S., & Park, K.-Y. (1994). Biochemical, microbiological, and nutritional aspects of kimchi (Korean fermented vegetable products). *Critical Reviews in Food Science and Nutrition*, 34(2), 175–203.

Chen, C., & Liu, B. Y. (2000). Changes in major components of tea fungus metabolites during prolonged fermentation. *Journal of Applied Microbiology*, 89(5), 834–839.

Cho, Y. R., Chang, J. Y., & Chang, H. C. (2007). Production of γ-aminobutyric acid (GABA) by Lactobacillus buchneri isolated from Kimchi and its neuroprotective effect on neuronal cells. *Journal of Microbiology and Biotechnology*, 17(1), 104–109.

De Filippis, F., Troise, A. D., Vitaglione, P., & Ercolini, D. (2018). Different temperatures select distinctive acetic acid bacteria species and promotes organic acids production during Kombucha tea fermentation. *Food Microbiology*, 73, 11–16.

Del Rio, D., Rodriguez-Mateos, A., Spencer, J. P. E., Tognolini, M., Borges, G., & Crozier, A. (2013). Dietary (Poly)phenolics in Human Health: Structures, Bioavailability, and Evidence of Protective Effects Against Chronic Diseases. *Antioxidants & Redox Signaling*, 18(14), 1818–1892.

Dufresne, C., & Farnworth, E. (2000). Tea, Kombucha, and health: A review. *Food Research International*, 33(6), 409–421.

Edmond, C. (2017). South Korean women will soon outlive us all. What's their secret? World Economic Forum. https://www.weforum.org/agenda/2017/07/south-korean-women-life-expectancy-kimchi/.

Eom, S. J., Hwang, J. E., Kim, H. S., Kim, K.-T., & Paik, H.-D. (2018). Anti-inflammatory and cytotoxic effects of ginseng extract bioconverted by Leuconostoc mesenteroides KCCM 12010P isolated from kimchi. *International Journal of Food Science & Technology*, 1–7.

Jayabalan, R., Malini, K., Sathishkumar, M., Swaminathan, K., & Yun, S.-E. (2010). Biochemical characteristics of tea fungus produced during kombucha fermentation. *Food Science and Biotechnology*, 19(3), 843–847.

Jeong, S. H., Lee, H. J., Jung, J. Y., Lee, S. H., Seo, H. Y., Park, W. S., & Jeon, C. O. (2013). Effects of red pepper powder on microbial communities and metabolites during kimchi fermentation. *International Journal of Food Microbiology*, 160(3), 252–259.

Ji Young Jung, Hee Lee, S., Myeong Kim, J., Su Park, M., Bae, J.-W., Hahn, Y., … Ok Jeon, C. (2011). Metagenomic Analysis of Kimchi, a Traditional Korean Fermented Food. *Applied and Environmental Microbiology*, 77(7), 2264–2274.

Jung, J. Y., Lee, S. H., Jin, H. M., Hahn, Y., Madsen, E. L., & Jeon, C. O. (2013). Metatranscriptomic analysis of lactic acid bacterial gene expression during kimchi fermentation. *International Journal of Food Microbiology*, 163(2–3), 171–179.

Jy, K., & Ey, C. (2016). Changes in Korean Adult Females' Intestinal Microbiota Resulting from Kimchi Intake. *Journal of Nutrition & Food Sciences*, 6(2).

Kallel, L., Desseaux, V., Hamdi, M., Stocker, P., & Ajandouz, E. H. (2012). Insights into the fermentation biochemistry of Kombucha teas and potential impacts of Kombucha drinking on starch digestion. *Food Research International*, 49(1), 226–232.

Kimchi and hypochondria keep South Koreans healthy. (2017). *Financial Times*. https://www.ft.com/content/63154cec-fa75-11e6-9516-2d969e0d3b65.

Klein, D. (2017). Can You Eat the Kombucha SCOBY? http://kombuchahome.com/can-eat-kombucha-scoby/ (accessed April 4, 2018).

Kontis, V., Bennett, J. E., Mathers, C. D., Li, G., Foreman, K., & Ezzati, M. (2017). Future life expectancy in 35 industrialised countries: projections with a Bayesian model ensemble. *Lancet* (London, England), 389(10076), 1323–1335.

Kwak, M. K., Liu, R., & Kang, S. O. (2018). Antimicrobial activity of cyclic dipeptides produced by Lactobacillus plantarum LBP-K10 against multidrug-resistant bacteria, pathogenic fungi, and influenza A virus. *Food Control*, 85, 223–234.

Kwon, M. (1997). Effects of kimchi on tissue and fecal lipid composition and apoprotein and thyroxine levels in rats. *J Korean Soc Food Sci Nutr*, 26, 507–513.

Lattimer, J. M., & Haub, M. D. (2010). Effects of Dietary Fiber and Its Components on Metabolic Health. *Nutrients*, 2(12), 1266–1289.

Lavasani, S., Dzhambazov, B., Nouri, M., Fåk, F., Buske, S., Molin, G., … Weström, B. (2010). A novel probiotic mixture exerts a therapeutic effect on experimental autoimmune encephalomyelitis mediated by IL-10 producing regulatory T cells. *PLoS ONE*, 5(2).

Lee, H., Yoon, H., Ji, Y., Kim, H., Park, H., Lee, J., ... Holzapfel, W. (2011). Functional properties of Lactobacillus strains isolated from kimchi. *International Journal of Food Microbiology*, 145(1), 155–161.

Lee, J. Y., Choi, M. K., & Kyung, K. H. (2008). Reappraisal of stimulatory effect of garlic on kimchi fermentation. *Korean Journal of Food Science and Technology*, 40(4), 479–484.

Lee, M., Song, J. H., Jung, M. Y., Lee, S. H., & Chang, J. Y. (2017). Large-scale targeted metagenomics analysis of bacterial ecological changes in 88 kimchi samples during fermentation. *Food Microbiology*, 66, 173–183.

Lee, S. H., Jung, J. Y., & Jeon, C. O. (2015). Source Tracking and Succession of Kimchi Lactic Acid Bacteria during Fermentation. *Journal of Food Science*, 80(8), M1871–M1877.

Lim, H. S., Cha, I. T., Roh, S. W., Shin, H. H., & Seo, M. J. (2017). Enhanced production of gamma-aminobutyric acid by optimizing culture conditions of Lactobacillus brevis HYE1 isolated from kimchi, a Korean fermented food. *Journal of Microbiology and Biotechnology*, 27(3), 450–459.

Malbaša, R., Lončar, E., Djurić, M., & Došenović, I. (2008). Effect of sucrose concentration on the products of Kombucha fermentation on molasses. *Food Chemistry*, 108(3), 926–932.

Malbaša, R., Lončar, E., Djurić, M., Klašnja, M., Kolarov, L. J., & Markov, S. (2006). Scale-up of black tea batch fermentation by Kombucha. *Food and Bioproducts Processing*, 84(3 C), 193–199.

Malbaša, R. V., Lončar, E. S., Vitas, J. S., & Čanadanović-Brunet, J. M. (2011). Influence of starter cultures on the antioxidant activity of kombucha beverage. *Food Chemistry*, 127(4), 1727–1731.

Malbaša, R. V., & Maksinovic, M. Z. (2004). The influence of starter cultures on the content of vitamin B2 in tea fungus beverages. *Central European Jounal of Occupational and Environmental Medicine*, 1, 79–83.

Marsh, A. J., O'Sullivan, O., Hill, C., Ross, R. P., & Cotter, P. D. (2014). Sequence-based analysis of the bacterial and fungal compositions of multiple kombucha (tea fungus) samples. *Food Microbiology*, 38, 171–178.



Nakakita, Y., Tsuchimoto, N., Takata, Y., & Nakamura, T. (2016). Effect of dietary heat-killed Lactobacillus brevis SBC8803 (SBL88TM) on sleep: A non-randomised, double blind, placebo-controlled, and crossover pilot study. *Beneficial Microbes*, 7(4), 501–509.

Neffe-Skocińska, K., Sionek, B., Ścibisz, I., & Kołożyn-Krajewska, D. (2017). Acid contents and the effect of fermentation condition of Kombucha tea beverages on physicochemical, microbiological and sensory properties. *CyTA - Journal of Food*, 15(4), 601–607.

Park, K.-Y., Jeong, J.-K., Lee, Y.-E., & Iii, J. W. D. (2014). Health Benefits of Kimchi (Korean Fermented Vegetables) as a Probiotic Food. *Journal of Medicinal Food*, 17(1), 6–20.

Park, S., Ji, Y., Park, H., Lee, K., Park, H., Beck, B. R., ... Holzapfel, W. H. (2016). Evaluation of functional properties of lactobacilli isolated from Korean white kimchi. *Food Control*, 69, 5–12.

Park, S., Kim, J. Il, Bae, J.-Y., Yoo, K., Kim, H., Kim, I.-H., ... Lee, I. (2018). Effects of heat-killed Lactobacillus plantarum against influenza viruses in mice. *Journal of Microbiology*, 56(2), 145–149.

Raymond, J. (2013). World's Healthiest Foods: Kimchi (Korea). *Health*. http://www.health.com/health/article/0,20410300,00.html.

Reva, O. N., Zaets, I. E., Ovcharenko, L. P., Kukharenko, O. E., Shpylova, S. P., Podolich, O. V, ... Kozyrovska, N. O. (2015). Metabarcoding of the kombucha microbial community grown in different microenvironments. *AMB Express*, 5(1).

Saikia, D., Kumar Manhar, A., Deka, B., Roy, R., Gupta, K., Namsa, N. D., ... Mandal, M. (2018). Hypocholesterolemic activity of indigenous probiotic isolate Saccharomyces cerevisiae ARDMC1 in a rat model. *Journal of Food and Drug Analysis*, 26, 154–162.

Saikia, D., Manhar, A. K., Deka, B., Roy, R., Gupta, K., Namsa, N. D., ... Mandal, M. (2018). Hypocholesterolemic activity of indigenous probiotic isolate Saccharomyces cerevisiae ARDMC1 in a rat model. *Journal of Food and Drug Analysis*, 26(1), 154–162.

Seo, B. J., Rather, I. A., Kumar, V. J. R., Choi, U. H., Moon, M. R., Lim, J. H., & Park, Y. H. (2012). Evaluation of Leuconostoc mesenteroides YML003 as a probiotic against low-pathogenic avian influenza (H9N2) virus in chickens. *Journal of Applied Microbiology*, 113(1), 163–171.

Seong, G.-U., Hwang, I.-W., & Chung, S.-K. (2016). Antioxidant capacities and polyphenolics of Chinese cabbage (Brassica rapa L. ssp. Pekinensis) leaves. *Food Chemistry*, 199, 612–618.

Son, S.-H., Jeon, H.-L., Jeon, E. B., Lee, N.-K., Park, Y.-S., Kang, D.-K., & Paik, H.-D. (2017). Potential probiotic Lactobacillus plantarum Ln4 from kimchi: Evaluation of β-galactosidase and antioxidant activities. *LWT - Food Science and Technology*, 85, 181–186.

Steenbergen, L., Sellaro, R., van Hemert, S., Bosch, J. A., & Colzato, L. S. (2015). A randomized controlled trial to test the effect of multispecies probiotics on cognitive reactivity to sad mood. *Brain, Behavior, and Immunity*, 48, 258–264.

Tamang, J. P. (2015). *Health Benefits of Fermented Foods and Beverages*. Boca Raton: CRC Press.

Teoh, A. L., Heard, G., & Cox, J. (2004). Yeast ecology of Kombucha fermentation. *International Journal of Food Microbiology*, 95(2), 119–126.

Vázquez-Cabral, B. D., Larrosa-Pérez, M., Gallegos-Infante, J. A., Moreno-Jiménez, M. R., González-Laredo, R. F., Rutiaga-Quiñones, J. G., ... Rocha-Guzmán, N. E. (2017). Oak kombucha protects against oxidative stress and inflammatory processes. *Chemico-Biological Interactions*, 272, 1–9.

Wang, K., Gan, X., Tang, X., Wang, S., & Tan, H. (2010). Determination of d-saccharic acid-1,4-lactone from brewed kombucha broth by high-performance capillary electrophoresis. *Journal of Chromatography B*, 878(3–4), 371–374.

Wen, L. S., Philip, K., & Ajam, N. (2016). Purification, characterization and mode of action of plantaricin K25 produced by Lactobacillus plantarum. *Food Control*, 60, 430–439.

Woo, M., Kim, M., Noh, J. S., Park, C. H., & Song, Y. O. (2018). Preventative activity of kimchi on high cholesterol diet-induced hepatic damage through regulation of lipid metabolism in LDL receptor knockout mice. *Food Science and Biotechnology*, 27(1), 211–218.

Xi, B., Veeranki, S. P., Zhao, M., Ma, C., Yan, Y., & Mi, J. (2017). Relationship of Alcohol Consumption to All-Cause, Cardiovascular, and Cancer-Related Mortality in U.S. Adults. *Journal of the American College of Cardiology*, 70(8), 913–922.

Yang, E. J., & Chang, H. C. (2010). Purification of a new antifungal compound produced by Lactobacillus plantarum AF1 isolated from kimchi. *International Journal of Food Microbiology*, 139(1–2), 56–63.

Yang, Z., Zhou, F., Ji, B., Li, B., Luo, Y., Yang, L., & Li, T. (2010). Symbiosis between Microorganisms from Kombucha and Kefir: Potential Significance to the Enhancement of Kombucha Function. *Applied Biochemistry and Biotechnology*, 160(2), 446–455.

Zamora-Ros, R., Rabassa, M., Cherubini, A., Urpí-Sardà, M., Bandinelli, S., Ferrucci, L., & Andres-Lacueva, C. (2013). High Concentrations of a Urinary Biomarker of Polyphenol Intake Are Associated with Decreased Mortality in Older Adults. *Journal of Nutrition*, 143(9), 1445–1450.

Zelman, K. (2017). Kombucha - Ingredients, Health Benefits, and Risks. https://www.webmd.com/diet/the-truth-about-kombucha (accessed April 4, 2018).

## CHAPTER 6

*TIME*. (2017). 13% of Americans Take Antidepressants. http://time.com/4900248/antidepressants-depression-more-common/.

# Index

# Thank You . . .

I'd like to start off by thanking everyone at Bonnier Fakta, my Swedish publisher, who, along with my publisher Cecilia Viklund at the helm, believed in me and my idea for this book. To write my first book with you has been one of the best (and hardest) things I have done. A huge thanks also goes out to Katy Kimbell, who designed the book with her magical illustrations. Together with Roland Persson's finely tuned photographs, they accompany the book perfectly. Most of all I want to thank my editor Linnéa von Zweigbergk, who helped me to weigh up each word carefully to make the book as readable as possible in the original Swedish language.

I also want to thank Karolinska Institute for equipping me with research skills; without my doctorate to back me up I would have probably not been able to review over four hundred scientific articles in such a short amount of time. A thank-you also goes out to all the competent researchers around the world (see the reference section, p. 177) whose work the book is based on. I hope I have done your work justice.

As this is a scientific book written for the average reader, I have obviously had to make some simplifications, and in light of the fact that this is a new and ever-changing research field, I used several fact-checkers. Therefore, a huge thank-you goes out to Johanna Sundin, Lina Tingö, Niclas Branzell, Nils Joneborg, and Fredrik Paulún.

I especially want to thank Johanna and Lina, who, with their in-depth knowledge on the gut-brain axis, provided many useful suggestions. A special thanks also goes to Niclas, who assisted me in different ways.

My good friend Magnus Brodén also receives a warm thanks for his support, and I also want to thank Seth Jacobs and his sister, Shawn Jacobs, who, on my daily walks around Boulder, Colorado, gave me tips on how to make your own kombucha.

My little mother, who has tirelessly cooked good Korean food and yummy kimchi during my whole writing process, gets a huge thank-you. Together we managed to visit the world's only kimchi museum, taste-test ourselves through Seoul, and experiment with a vast range of kimchi types with Aunt Jinju—all to get the best kimchi recipes for the book. Thanks, Mom!

Last but not least, I want to thank my little brother, Sung-Kyu Choi, and his wife, Carola Choi, who are always there, like a warm blanket, whenever I need them. This book is dedicated to your wonderful daughters Ella and Esther, who make life more colorful and the future of health more positive. Without our crazy adventures and games with Pruski, the writing process would have been a lot harder. Thank you for being there!

If you want to join in on the exciting research on how bacteria can strengthen your brain, or just be inspired by more brain-friendly recipes, you can visit me at www.sokichoi.com.

# Conversion Charts

## Metric and Imperial Conversions

(These conversions are rounded for convenience)

| Ingredient | Cups/Tablespoons/ Teaspoons | Ounces | Grams/Milliliters |
|---|---|---|---|
| Butter | 1 cup/ 16 tablespoons/ 2 sticks | 8 ounces | 230 grams |
| Cheese, shredded | 1 cup | 4 ounces | 110 grams |
| Cream cheese | 1 tablespoon | 0.5 ounce | 14.5 grams |
| Cornstarch | 1 tablespoon | 0.3 ounce | 8 grams |
| Flour, all-purpose | 1 cup/1 tablespoon | 4.5 ounces/0.3 ounce | 125 grams/8 grams |
| Flour, whole wheat | 1 cup | 4 ounces | 120 grams |
| Fruit, dried | 1 cup | 4 ounces | 120 grams |
| Fruits or veggies, chopped | 1 cup | 5 to 7 ounces | 145 to 200 grams |
| Fruits or veggies, pureed | 1 cup | 8.5 ounces | 245 grams |
| Honey, maple syrup, or corn syrup | 1 tablespoon | 0.75 ounce | 20 grams |
| Liquids: cream, milk, water, or juice | 1 cup | 8 fluid ounces | 240 milliliters |
| Oats | 1 cup | 5.5 ounces | 150 grams |
| Salt | 1 teaspoon | 0.2 ounce | 6 grams |
| Spices: cinnamon, cloves, ginger, or nutmeg (ground) | 1 teaspoon | 0.2 ounce | 5 milliliters |
| Sugar, brown, firmly packed | 1 cup | 7 ounces | 200 grams |
| Sugar, white | 1 cup/1 tablespoon | 7 ounces/0.5 ounce | 200 grams/12.5 grams |
| Vanilla extract | 1 teaspoon | 0.2 ounce | 4 grams |



## Oven Temperatures

| Fahrenheit | Celsius | Gas Mark |
|---|---|---|
| 225° | 110° | 1/4 |
| 250° | 120° | 1/2 |
| 275° | 140° | 1 |
| 300° | 150° | 2 |
| 325° | 160° | 3 |
| 350° | 180° | 4 |
| 375° | 190° | 5 |
| 400° | 200° | 6 |
| 425° | 220° | 7 |
| 450° | 230° | 8 |